Théodore Potter

Essays on bacteriology and its relation to the progress of medicine

Theodore Potter

Essays on bacteriology and its relation to the progress of medicine

ISBN/EAN: 9783742827456

Manufactured in Europe, USA, Canada, Australia, Japan

Cover: Foto ©Lupo / pixelio.de

Manufactured and distributed by brebook publishing software
(www.brebook.com)

Théodore Potter

Essays on bacteriology and its relation to the progress of medicine

ESSAYS ON BACTERIOLOGY

AND ITS

RELATION TO THE PROGRESS OF MEDICINE

BY

THEODORE POTTER, A. M., M. D.

1 4

PROFESSOR OF PATHOLOGY AND BACTERIOLOGY IN THE MEDICAL COLLEGE OF INDIANA,
INDIANAPOLIS UNIVERSITY; MEMBER OF CONSULTING STAFF, CITY HOSPITAL AND
THE DEACONESS HOSPITAL; CONSULTING PHYSICIAN FOR DISEASES
OF THE CHEST, INDIANAPOLIS CITY DISPENSARY

THE INDIANA MEDICAL JOURNAL PUBLISHING COMPANY
INDIANAPOLIS
1898

DEDICATION

CONTENTS

PREFACE

————

This publication is the outgrowth of work done for the Indiana profession, having its origin in a series of papers upon the progress of bacteriology presented, by request, to the State Medical Society between the years 1890 and 1897.

These papers cover much of the time during which the germ theory of disease was working its way into the convictions of the profession, and it is with some little pride that the author is enabled to feel that of this progress he has been a part.

Presented under the special conditions indicated, and in serial form, they have something of a historical character and meaning which, even at the expense of some repetitions, has been in large measure preserved.

To these have been added several, partly new, partly prepared for the students of the Medical College of Indiana or for various medical gatherings.

Those numbered from 2 to 8 in the Table of Contents are given in the order of their preparation, covering the years 1890 to 1896.

I am indebted to Dr. E. D. Clark and Dr. C. E. Ferguson for aid in revising the manuscript, and to Dr. A. W. Brayton for constant encouragement and assistance in the preparation and arrangement of the book.

Should the presentation of these essays in book form be as kindly received by others as most of them have already been by my friends, the doctors of Indiana, it will be all that the author can ask.

INDIANAPOLIS,
    February, 1898.

ESSAYS ON BACTERIOLOGY

I.

THE GERM THEORY OF DISEASE.

THE germ theory of disease, now no longer a theory, but a demonstration of science, is a very simple doctrine. It asserts that certain disorders are due to the presence and growth, in the body, of living poisons called microbes, germs, bacteria, and that without such bacteria these diseases do not exist. Notice that certain disorders are said to have this origin; for no one asserts or supposes that all diseases are caused by bacteria. It is the maladies belonging to the group called infectious which are due to living agents, chief among which are the microscopic fungi now commonly known as bacteria or germs. This statement is a sufficient answer to the question, often asked, whether we believe all diseases to be due to microbes.

And here we notice two interesting and important facts growing out of bacteriology. The first is that the revelations of bacteriology have altered the classification of diseases, increasing the number of those included among the infections. Thus, the discovery of the germ of diphtheria has resulted in establishing the fact that so-called membranous croup is usually laryngeal diphtheria, and is therefore to be looked upon as an infectious disease. A similar thing is true of pneumonia, and notably of tuberculosis, over the character and classification of which a controversy was waged. We now know that tuberculosis is an infectious disease; a half-century ago this was only surmise.

We have learned, too, as a result of bacteriological studies, more of the importance of infection as an indirect cause of suffering and death. Thus, while we do not consider apoplexy an infectious disease, we have come to see more and more clearly that, in the last analysis, it is frequently a product of infection. The blood vessels of the brain do not break unless they are injured or diseased, and the disease which thus makes a cerebral apoplexy possible is often of infectious character or the indirect result of an infection. It matters not that this indirect result is sometimes seen only after many years: the fact remains, and must constantly be borne in mind in practical medicine. The man who falls by an apoplectic stroke often falls from an infectious blow struck years before, perhaps when sowing the proverbial wild oats of youth. And thus one may literally reap a harvest of death from seeds sown and long since forgotten.

Thus we learn, notwithstanding the charge sometimes brought that the germ theory of disease is made to account for too much, that its field of action is really wider than is commonly supposed. As we look about us and see the havoc wrought, directly and indirectly, we may fairly say that it is hardly possible to exaggerate the importance of infection and of the minute agents which produce it. The invisible enemies are here, as elsewhere, the most numerous and dangerous.

The germ theory of disease is no new thing. Though it has but recently come into prominence, and its truth but recently been demonstrated, it is, as a theory, as old, almost, as history. Crude, ill-defined, and as crudely expressed, it has nevertheless been for ages essentially the same. Hippocrates saw and believed in it; and from his day to ours it has served as a rallying cry for warring factions and for the disputes of the learned. At times it has assumed prominence, through the influence of some master mind great in its capacity to grasp a simple and far-reaching truth. Again it has sunk almost into oblivion, carried down by the weight of its own artificially and ignorantly imposed absurdities. Thus it has risen and fallen, come and gone, with the varying tide of speculative fashion. In this unstable but enduring history there must be some reason, and for it we have not far to look.

We can readily see why the germ theory of disease so persistently suggested and asserted itself to men's minds. They saw many of the facts which we see. They saw a small amount of poison enter the body of

an animal or man, and afterward that the body contained a much larger quantity of the poison. They
saw one case of a disease enter a community, and
afterward they saw, with strong evidence of transfer
from one to another, that many others had the disease.
From such facts they made the same inference as we
do. They said: these poisons seem to grow and multiply; they must be living; for such properties as true
growth and reproduction they, as we, only knew as belonging to living things. And this is the germ theory
of disease. When we inquire why this simple and
logical doctrine became, at times, contaminated with
so much absurdity as to bring it into merited discredit
and to even threaten its survival, the answer is not
difficult to find.

However rational, however logical, it was but a
theory, a mere speculation, shrouded in mystery. The
ignorant mind loves mystery, and all men love to
speculate about that which they cannot prove. We
all love to peer into the darkness, and where we cannot see we quickly bring imagination into play. A
Greek proverb tells us that the mysterious is always
great, and imaginary greatness is easily distorted into
absurdity. It is as true in medicine as in theology
that men often make the most positive and at the
same time most extravagant assertions about things of
which they know the least.

Thus the germ theory of disease became at times so
distorted, the subject of so many evidently unwar-

ranted embellishments, that honestly ignorant men refused to believe it.

When we inquire why, aside from such abuses, this rational and simple explanation of the infectious diseases remained so long a mere theory, the answer, in the light of present knowledge, is again not difficult. "Knowledge is of things we see," and there were no means of seeing these minute objects which, with so much reason, were supposed to exist. It was only after the microscope, the aid to vision, was so far perfected as to enable men to look upon bacteria that it could be demonstrated that such things really existed. And only after many years of gradual improvement of this wonderful instrument was this obstacle to progress overcome.

But to see bacteria in disease, even to prove by observation their constant presence, is not sufficient to demonstrate their causative influence. It can at best prove only that they are regularly associated with abnormal processes in the body, and furnish strong evidence that they are living beings. If now we will go a step further and prove that they are actually the seeds of disease, we must do what the agriculturist does. We must be able to handle these seeds, to separate them from one another, to sort out the different varieties, to obtain these varieties in sufficient quantity for experiment; we must be able to plant them, follow their growth, and find out what that growth will produce. We must, in a word, cultivate these our disease seeds as the agriculturist does his.

This now we are able to do. We can see bacteria, can cultivate them, can identify and grow the different varieties. We can plant them in the bodies of men and animals, and reproduce at will the diseases from which the bacteria were obtained. And thus we are able to prove our theory. It is the invention of methods for the artificial cultivation of bacteria which has made it possible for us to handle and work with these minute organisms, and which, with the aid of the microscope, has removed the germ theory of disease from the realm of speculation and established it, as I have said, as a demonstration of science.

The germ theory of disease is no longer matter of dispute. It is as clearly demonstrated as the laws of gravitation. Of him who does not know it it is to be said that he has not as yet really heard the evidence in the case. If anyone is still held in the bondage of doubt, he has but to hear with an open ear this evidence, and he will know the truth. And this truth will make him free.

II.

SOME OF THE PROBLEMS OF BACTERIOLOGY.

THERE is no subject which, during the last decade, has occupied as large a part of the attention and interest of the profession as the germ theory of disease. It is perhaps safe to say that it would have been impossible during the last few years to find a single issue of any medical journal in Europe or America which did not contain some reference to it. It is also safe to say that the medical historian of the future will describe our age as chiefly characterized by the developments in this direction, and that, in the word picture, the germ theory of disease will stand out pre-eminent.

When we consider the large proportion of suffering and death due to the infectious diseases, medical and surgical, and remember that this theory has offered an explanation of their causation, propagation and many of their phenomena, and points to methods not only of cure, but of prevention, which is greater than cure, we are not surprised that it should have risen rapidly into prominence and already exercised such an influence in medical thought and action.

The rise of the germ theory of disease, as we now
know it, is one of those great movements—wide, deep
and far-reaching, such as are seen only now and then
in the progress of medicine, and which stamp the
character of its succeeding generations. It has modified and advanced our ideas of etiology; it has entered
the field of pathology and wrought great changes in
it, so that, for instance, we now say, in the language
of Strumpel: "The definition of tuberculosis has
now removed itself from a merely anatomical basis; it
is that disease which is called forth by the active
agency of the tubercle bacillus."   Dr. Senn has recently expressed the opinion, the truth of which I
neither deny nor affirm, that "more real progress has
been made in surgical pathology during the last fifteen years than in twenty centuries preceding," and
that "surgical pathology has become almost synony-
mous with surgical bacteriology." Though to a limited extent, yet distinctly and helpfully, it has increased our diagnostic abilities; it has added something to medical treatment, and has aroused, stimu-
lated, and guided many earnest efforts in this direction. It has strengthened the safeguards about the
puerperal woman, and so modified the methods of surgery and emboldened its practice as to add much to
its efficiency. It has entered the broad realm of sanitary science and preventive medicine, and, throwing a
new ray of light toward that promised land, has
brightened our hopes for the coming of a better day.

Bacteriology has passed the stage of curiosity and sensation; it is not a scientific by-play nor a microscopic diversion; it is a study of pathology and the causation of disease, and as such has taken its place among the branches of medical science and in the curriculum of medical studies. We are all watching it—interested in it, and now that it has become a somewhat old story, must often ask ourselves: What is it doing and what does it propose to do? What problems are before it and how is it endeavoring to solve these problems?

Laying aside mere details and technicalities, which, after all, attract the intelligent mind the least, I have thought it might be of interest to consider very briefly some of those problems which have been engaging the attention of workers in this line, problems arising in the struggle to overcome obstacles to the further development of the work, problems involved in the effort to render practically valuable the results already reached. Omitting some which are of much, perhaps of equal, importance, I mention the following:

Questions of the susceptibility of animals to the infectious diseases; the durability of infectious material; of disinfection; the manner of dissemination of disease germs; are all infectious diseases due to one specific cause; the question of hereditary transmission.

Koch lays down four postulates which must be satisfied before we can fully accept the causative relation between a bacterium and a disease. The last two of these refer to inoculation; and the inoculation experiments are the final and crucial tests of bacteriology, at least so far as the pathogenic character of the organisms is concerned. But here a difficulty is at once met. It is evidently impossible to inoculate men with the supposed causes of such diseases as cholera, tuberculosis, typhoid, syphilis, anthrax and glanders. Animals must therefore be used, and the question must at once be answered: are animals susceptible to all the infectious diseases? This question resolves itself into two: are they susceptible, and how do the diseases manifest themselves? By what signs and lesions may we know that an animal suffers from or dies of a certain disease? Are we to expect the same symptoms and lesions as are found in human beings? If not, they must be studied out for animals as they have been for man.

The susceptibility of animals to certain infections is easily recognized; for instance, to erysipelas, suppuration, tuberculosis, anthrax, glanders and others. Some animals are apparently entirely refractory to one or more diseases to which others are very sensitive. Moreover, it is not sufficient merely to show that inoculation with pure cultures will kill an animal; it may have died of a sapremia or septicemia, not of a specific disease from which the organism was obtained. For there are organisms which are not known to have a constant causative relation to any specific disease, which, nevertheless, will produce pronounced toxic effects when inoculated.

To illustrate the difficulties in this matter: It was at first found that feeding with cultures of the comma bacillus of cholera would not injure animals. The result was, great doubt and even ridicule thrown upon it. Some skeptics even offered to swallow any quantity themselves. These facts are fresh in the minds of all. But the comma bacillus flourishes in an alkaline medium, and, following up this indication, it was found that inoculation directly into the duodenum gave very pronounced results. Finally, after washing the stomach, injecting a sterile alkaline solution, lessening peristalsis by opium, and then feeding or injecting through a tube, the comma bacilli show themselves any thing but the harmless beings once supposed.

It is well known that an organism has been identified in connection with typhoid fever and is generally supposed to be the cause of that disease. But it is still uncertain. Koch himself has recently, I believe, taken this position, that while the Koch-Eberth bacillus is probably the specific germ, the final demonstration has not yet been reached. The reason of this uncertainty is the unsatisfactory character of the inoculation experiments. For it is not yet known whether animals are subject to this disease; they may die from the artificial infection, but it is not certain that a group of symptoms and lesions can be identified in them, constituting the specific disease typhoid fever.

2

This question, then, of the relation of animals to the infectious diseases is evidently one of importance in bacteriological investigations, and the uncertainties connected with it furnish an obstacle which is often deplored. Obviously also, as the work progresses, here must open fields for painstaking and interesting research. Incidentally these researches may throw a valuable light upon veterinary medicine.

Is each of the infectious diseases due to a single and constant, a specific cause? From the evident uniformity in their phenomena, it is generally believed that this is true; and, for most of them at least, the supposition is in all probability correct. Yet there are some facts which have seemed to throw doubt upon this belief, and in its present condition bacteriology cannot answer the question with absolute certainty. Two organisms, for instance, have been identified in connection with croupous pneumonia; that of Fried-lander, and the Sternberg-Pasteur-Fraenkel micrococcus. It is claimed that by inoculation with each of these a more or less typical exudative inflammation of the lungs has been produced. But they do not satisfy the postulates of Koch. Neither has been found constantly in pneumonia, and both have been found under other conditions. So true is this that Fraenkel has called one of them the microbe of sputum septicaemia rather than of pneumonia. A similar condition of uncertainty exists in the bacteriology of diphtheria.

Such experimental results as these, even though

there still be much doubt about them, at least raise the question whether some of the supposed infectious diseases may not be due to more than one cause; whether, to put it concretely, an acute, self-limited, croupous inflammation of the lungs, such as characterizes pneumonia, or such lesions as belong to diphtheria, may not be produced by more than one agent. Probably not; yet it must be said that recent bacteriological work has opened the question and has left it still open.

Allied to this is the interesting inquiry whether a pathogenic micro-organism may, in different localities, and under different conditions, produce apparently different diseases. A connection between erysipelas and puerperal fever has long been suspected, and recent research has strengthened this suspicion. Various authorities have asserted, on the basis of experiment, that the Fehleisen streptococcus of erysipelas would produce puerperal fever, and that the streptococcus often found in the latter disease would produce erysipelas. Some believe, partly because of these facts, and partly because of the close resemblance in the organisms, that they are the same. Certain it seems, however, that an organism which would produce erysipelas has a number of times been cultivated from child-bed fever.

The question of the durability of infectious material is one which has long interested and often puzzled the profession. It is not strange that it should

have been almost constantly under discussion, for it
confronts us daily, as practicing physicians, and is of
great importance in the broader sphere of preventive
medicine. To illustrate: When may children re-
turn to school from a family in which an infectious
disease has been prevailing? If tuberculosis is an infectious disease, how long does tuberculous matter remain dangerous?

It would not be at all true nor fair to say that all
our present knowledge on this subject has come from
bacteriology; far from it. Much of it is the result of
that painstaking observation and study which pre-
vailed in former days. But much is the product of
the last few years; and in this connection it is to be
noted that progress of late has been upon more definite lines. If the infectious diseases are due to living
things, this question resolves itself chiefly into a study
of those organisms. A specific germ being identified,
the question, how long may the poison of this disease
continue as poison, becomes, how long may this germ
live? The investigation evidently centers at once
upon a more definite point. How long, then, may
bacteria live? The answer is: it depends upon certain
conditions; and it is the discovery of the germs themselves, and increasing knowledge of the conditions
upon which their life depends, which has brought us
closer to a solution of this problem.

The life and growth of bacteria depends upon the
soil on which they are placed, and the external influ-

ences to which they are subjected. Two groups of factors have, therefore, been studied in the effort to obtain more definite knowledge of the durability of infectious material, that is, the tenacity of life of micro-organisms. Elaborate investigations have been made of the relation between various bacteria and the media containing them, and thus has opened up a large field for the study of the growth and durability of bacteria in various food substances, in milk and in water. Thus, in milk many find a congenial home; in water some retain their vitality for a long time, others soon disappear. But aside from culture soils, certain conditions have much to do with the life-history of bacteria, the most important being temperature, moisture, and the presence or absence of air. Some grow only at high temperatures, that is, at about body-heat; others at a much lower point. Some retain life in the absence of any notable amount of moisture, others quickly die when dried. Some grow only in the presence of air, others flourish without it, and hence the division into aerobic and anaerobic bacteria.

Then, too, considerable study has been made of the destiny of bacteria in the body after death. The results are not as yet very conclusive, but the weight of evidence seems to be that many kinds of germs soon disappear. Esmarch has recently gone over this ground again, his conclusion being that just stated; an inference being that graveyards are not as dangerous as has been supposed.

Without following the details of this subject further, it may be said that our ideas of the durability of infectious material have become more definite, the lines of investigation have been much more sharply defined, additions of much practical value have been made to our knowledge, and we have reason to expect more light in the near future. To illustrate what has been done: It has been shown that the gonorrheal poison rapidly loses its virulence; after even a short period of drying outside the body it can neither be cultivated nor inoculated. On the other hand, the ordinary pus germs have been found to be very tenacious of life. Rosenbach, to whom we owe most of our knowledge of them, has found them active after two years in a culture tube.

But far and away beyond anything in this line is the discovery that the essential infecting agent in tuberculous material may maintain its vitality for months, even in a dried state, and not only its vitality, but also its malevolent infectious character. Upon this fact is based one of the most important discussions which is at present agitating the medical and sanitary world.

Closely connected with this problem of the durability of infectious material is the question: How and by what channels is it carried? Here, again, a large part of our knowledge antedates bacteriology. But the older methods were difficult, slow, and often uncertain, and not infrequently, while furnishing most valuable facts, left them without satisfactory explanation. I have already emphasized the fact that bacteriology has placed this and kindred investigations upon a more secure foundation; has laid down the lines more sharply, and given to means and methods a more definite aim. How this is true must be evident. A definite material thing having become known as the essential infecting agent, the methods of its identification, its life-history and the conditions of its durability established, we at once know what to search for in the endeavor to trace the poison from place to place or person to person. Thus earth, air, water, foods, hands, instruments, fomites of various kinds, are made to yield their secrets, and are known as, not hypothetical, but proven carriers of disease. To draw illustration again from the great scourge: If it be shown that the tubercle bacillus is the sinning agent in the tuberculous material, that it exists in the products of the lesions, that it retains its vitality through long periods under apparently adverse conditions, that it can be detected in its hiding places outside the body, and, with virulence unchanged, can be traced through milk, clothing, furniture, floors and dust; if these things are true, is it to be wondered at that they have modified the older opinions, and are leading many to believe that we have come nearer to a solution of one of the medical riddles of the ages?

Among all the subjects which might be brought under the title of this paper there is, perhaps, nothing

more striking than the contrast between disinfection
before and since the recent growth of bacteriology.
Heretofore it has been in some respects almost like
beating the air or fighting in the dark. Now the general problem of disinfection has reduced itself to this:
How most efficiently and with least danger to insure
the destruction of disease germs. The second condition is important because many germicidal agents are
active poisons.

Definite knowledge having been reached as to just
what is to be destroyed, experimenters are at once
able to drive at the heart of the first problem of disinfection: What agents will destroy these bacteria,
and what is their relative germicidal power? As the
result of these studies, bi-chloride of mercury stands
at the head of chemical agents, heat of the non-chem-
ical; and perhaps the most important result of the investigation of disinfectants is the high place given to
heat, not only in theory but in practice.

Another interesting and important set of facts has
been brought out, as the result of which disinfectants
have been classified, as to their activity, as follows:
First, those which rapidly destroy both bacteria and
spores; second, those which destroy mature bacteria
but not spores; third, those which prevent the development of bacteria or spores, and, finally, those which
more or less retard their development. It will at once
be seen that this classification is of more than theoretical interest. For, as is well known, many if not all of

the chemical germicides are poisons. Their use therefore to the point of destruction of the bacteria might also result in destruction of the host. Obstetricians have learned this by some bitter experiences. It is therefore a matter of very practical value to know that below the point of lethal strength these agents may prevent, or so far retard the growth of bacteria as to make their action truly disinfectant. It is well to remember this, that it is not an irrational nor a useless thing to use weak solutions of disinfectants.

Another point which has been made clear is, that the relative practical value of these agents is not the same as their relative germicidal power, and that the strongest germicide is not necessarily always the best to use. This fact rests not solely upon the poisonous quality of some of the chemical disinfectants, but upon other grounds also. Thus, the bi-chloride of mercury, in the presence of albumen, is thrown down as an insoluble albumenate. This everyone has seen in dressing a bleeding wound. Solutions of this substance, even when made with ordinary distilled water of the shops, may be much weaker than their users innocently believe. Hence, the plan of adding such agents as ammonium chloride or tartaric acid to prevent this change. Other things of minor importance are also to be taken into account in deciding the question of the practical utility of germicides, as their irritant, corrosive, or staining properties, their cost, odor, solubility, etc.

When we come to consider the question of disinfection of such substances as clothing, bedding, sputa and feces, it is evident that we are in a much better position to do effective work than our predecessors. We no longer confound deodorants and disinfectants. Every one who has read "The Innocents Abroad" will remember the picture of the unfortunate passengers, just landed from their ship, undergoing the horrible and probably quite useless fumigation. There is more than a suspicion that the deodorant properties of the sulphur were mistaken for disinfectant virtues. We smile at it now, but it was an honest effort.

Do we wish to know how best to disinfect a bale of rags from Italy? The bacteriological test is comparatively simple and certain. What method will render tuberculous sputum harmless? The test is the same. Will we learn how to purify the materials from a sick room? Look for the effect upon the agents of infection. The verdict over the pestiferous intruders: "Dead, for a ducat, dead," is worth more than all the odors which sulphurous compounds can emit.

The intimate relation between bacteriology and the question of the hereditary transmission of disease becomes at once evident if the truth of the recent ideas as to the cause of the infections diseases be admitted. If bacteria are the sole exciting cause of certain diseases, if these maladies cannot exist without their agency, then the hereditary transmission of such diseases means the transmission from parent to offspring of these bacteria. This by no means rules out the existence and importance of predisposing causes, but it brings the chief and most direct factor into the foreground, and limits the investigation to a narrower, more definite and more pointed question.

Do bacteria or their spores pass from parent to offspring with the beginning of or during intra-uterine life? Does the fetus emerge from its mother's uterus with the germs in its body? The light on this question of heredity has heretofore come chiefly from a clinical rather than a pathological source. An immense mass of clinical facts has been gathered, but has not sufficed to settle the whole matter. Notably is this uncertainty true of tuberculosis, that disease in connection with which the study of heredity is of such importance. Many cases have been recorded which seem to prove that certain infections diseases may be transmitted to the fetus, as smallpox and measles. Further, it seems to have been shown that the bacilli of anthrax may pass from the mother to the young in utero. We have, then, apparent proof of hereditary transmission of an infections disease whose bacteria, if such exist, are not known, and of one with whose bacteria we are thoroughly acquainted. It seems, therefore, not unreasonable to suppose, the supposition being strengthened by the well-known clinical facts, that such a disease as tuberculosis may be acquired before birth. Parties are divided on this question, some holding the opinion expressed by Whittaker,

that the supposed hereditary acquisition of tuberculosis resolves itself into the results of association of
cases, in other words, post-natal infection. Others
hold to the view which commonly prevails; while
some endeavor to explain the facts upon the theory, of
which Baumgarten is the chief exponent, that the
bacilli received by heredity often remain latent for
months or years, springing into activity with the rise
of conditions favorable to their growth. Evidently,
more light must be obtained before the problem can
be solved, and bacteriology has stepped in with an
offer of aid; first, by showing what is the actual cause
of the disease, and leading in the search for this definite material thing in the body of the fetus. The
greatest interest has centered around tuberculosis, for
obvious reasons.

I do not propose to enter here into elaborate details,
but simply to indicate the lines along which the investigations have run. The search has been made by
microscopic examinations, by cultivations, and by inoculation experiments. Thus, a number of female
animals are inoculated with tuberculosis. They are
bred, if not already pregnant. Only the fetuses of
such mothers as can be proven to have the disease are
used. Their bodies being carefully protected from
contamination, the following experiments are made
upon them: They are examined microscopically, cultures are made from them and portions of their bodies
are inoculated into healthy animals. The cultures

and inoculations are made in order that if the bacteria should escape ocular detection they may still be found. On the strength of these researches some have claimed to prove the passage of the germs to the fetus, while some, conducting their studies with every precaution, have reached only negative results, and have believed that the apparent exceptions in the hands of others were due to contamination. A report made to the Paris Academy about a year ago was entirely negative, and this has been the rule. The well-known case of Johne, who proved fetal tuberculosis in a calf, stands alone unquestioned.

The end has not yet been reached. There are still claims and counter-claims, strong beliefs and influential skepticism. Certainly some of the infectious diseases seem to be transmitted by heredity, or at least to be congenital. As regards tuberculosis, there has been an unmistakable growth of the opinion that the disease is to be looked upon as an infection, not an inheritance: that the ideas of its heredity have been much exaggerated; that it is comparatively rarely transmitted to the fetus—perhaps never. How much of the hopes of preventive medicine depend upon the truth of these opinions is at once apparent. Whether we shall fail to reach positive knowledge, and, opinion wavering, the pendulum shall swing again toward its former position, remains to be seen. In the meantime let us get a clear view of the facts already established, give due credit and appreciation to the sincere and earnest efforts for the solution of the great ques-

tion, and, as practicing physicians, not forget the facts
of clinical experience.

I have not in this paper discussed nor raised the
question of the truth or falsity of the germ theory of
disease, nor entered further than was necessary into
the details and technicalities of bacteriology. I have
purposely avoided these things in order that I might
insist upon the idea that they are of secondary interest. Bacteriology is a study of pathology and the
causation of disease, and of the problems which gather
about these two great fields in medicine. It is only
as we thus think of it that we shall be able to understand what it is and what it means.

Though we are, and must be first of all, practitioners of medicine, it is well for us now and then to stop
and think what some of these things mean and where
we stand upon some of the great problems which are
arising in our profession; to think whence we have
come, and why, and whither we are going. Surely,
if we preserve our balance aright, it need not make us
less efficient actors if we keep ourselves somewhat in
touch with the world of theory and of thought.

If this discussion shall have succeeded in some degree in throwing the laboratory, the microscope and
the more details of bacteriology into the background,
and in placing in deserved prominence some of those
living problems which should most interest the intelligent physician, should attract his attention, enlist his
sympathy and engage his thought, its object will have
been accomplished.

III.

SPECIFIC DISEASES AND SPECIFIC BACTERIA.

AS practicing physicians we are always interested in the question: What is the status of our knowledge of the relation between individual diseases and specific bacteria? In other words: What do we now know of the specific causes of the infectious diseases?

It is not my intention to review the whole field, but confining myself to the more important diseases which affect mankind, to endeavor to answer the question: What do we know of their germ origin?

It cannot be said that any striking discoveries of new disease-producing germs have been made of late; but much has been done in solving some vexed questions and in clearing up some uncertain points.

During the first few years after the new methods had come into use, and under the stimulus of the epoch-making work of Koch and Pasteur, discoveries came thick and fast. Indeed, it almost seemed as though one could not gain repute in bacteriology without first having attached his name to some new germ. Of late years progress in this line has been

slower, the discovery of new bacteria has become
of less importance. The germ theory of disease has
been absolutely established, the specific germs of certain infectious diseases have apparently been settled,
and there is a general agreement as to the probable
bacterial origin of the others whose specific germs are
not yet known. The grounds for this belief are well
understood and need not be reviewed here.

The question is often asked why the bacteria of certain diseases, as measles and scarlatina, which are common enough and are evidently infectious, have not
been discovered. There is, of course, every reason to
believe that these maladies are due to living poisons,
and it does seem strange that they have thus far
baffled investigation. The more strange does it seem
at first sight, in view of the fact that the methods of
bacteriological research are now so well understood
and the cultivation of many germs so comparatively
easy.

There are, however, some marked differences between the poisons of measles, scarlatina, smallpox,
and many other infectious diseases. For instance,
they are apparently much more readily disseminated
through the air; they are said to be more "volatile."
The opinion, therefore, has grown that these differences are indicators of others more profound, and
which make it impossible to cultivate them by the ordinary methods. Until, therefore, further progress
has been made and perhaps radically new methods in-

troduced, it is possible that the bacteria of these diseases may remain in obscurity. There are other difficulties in the way of the investigations, some of which have already been explained. The problems are not as simple and easy of solution as some suppose; and we could hardly expect that, in the few years since modern bacteriology arose, the field would have been swept clean and there remain no more undiscovered territory.

Turning now from this explanation, let us review briefly our knowledge of the specific bacterial causes of the infectious diseases, remembering that with some the demonstration seems to be complete, with others only a high degree of probability has been reached; with many there is still a large element of uncertainty.

In making this summary I shall omit such facts as are already commonly known, and shall divide the diseases into several classes:

First. Those of which it may be said that the question of their bacterial origin is apparently settled. It will, perhaps, be surprising to some that so few are included in this class. They are anthrax, tuberculosis, glanders, suppuration, tetanus, erysipelas. Probably more increase in knowledge has of late come in regard to tetanus than any other of the diseases included in this group. The mystery in regard to this grave affection has apparently been cleared up. Kitasato has succeeded in perfecting a method of producing pure cultures, and by repeatedly successful inoculation experiments removed all doubt as to the fons et origo mali. The tetanus bacillus is a large rod, rounded at the ends, sometimes growing to long threads. It is motile, grows at ordinary temperature, and is strictly anaerobic—i. e., it does not grow in contact with the oxygen of the air. It stains easily by the ordinary methods. It is found in garden mould, on walls, in putrefying fluids, in manure, and in places frequented by horses. The association of tetanus bacilli with the earth and with horses has been strongly insisted on by a number of investigators. It is a striking fact that the bacilli are not found distributed through the body after death, and that their number at the point of infection is not proportional to the severity of the symptoms. This is explained by the discovery that the bacilli give rise to a most virulent poison, which, freed from germs, is capable of producing death with all the symptoms of the disease. The anaerobic quality of the germ probably explains the fact that penetrating wounds are especially liable to be followed by tetanus.

As to erysipelas, authorities are agreed that the same germ causes both traumatic and so-called idiopathic erysipelas. The sharp line hitherto drawn between these varieties of the disease should therefore be removed.

In regard to the bacilli of tuberculosis, some interesting investigations have been made in several directions.

First. It seems to have been shown by Ernst and others that the bacilli may be present and living in the milk of cows whose udders are not tuberculous. The importance of this fact will at once be recognized.

Second. A series of experiments has been carried out to decide whether the bacilli could penetrate the apparently healthy mucous membrane. The result is the conclusion that they can, together with the discovery that they are, under such circumstances, likely to be caught in the nearest lymph glands, and may produce the phenomena of ordinary tuberculous adenitis. These investigations are held to throw light upon the character of so-called scrofula.

Third. The immensely important question of latent tuberculosis appears to be nearing a solution, inasmuch as it has been shown that the bronchial and other glands of apparently healthy persons may contain living tubercle bacilli, and this, too, in the absence of any visible tuberculous lesions. H. P. Loomis has recently recorded a series of autopsies confirming this statement. If it be shown that long latent tuberculosis may exist in the body, or that bacilli may remain in the body through long periods without producing the disease, it will at once be seen how this fact will explain many things in the clinical history of the disease, and how it may throw light on the still vexed question of hereditary transmission. As to the hereditary transmission of tuberculosis, the investigations are still going on, but a certain conclusion has not been reached. The establishment of the possibility of bacilli remaining long inactive in the body has given the advocates of heredity, of whom Baumgarten is the leader, a firmer ground for their belief. In addition to the case of Johne, a few more of hereditary transmission in animals have been recorded, and, it is claimed, one in man. Were I asked to express an opinion upon this matter, I would almost repeat my former words: that there is a growing belief that the older ideas of heredity are exaggerated; that the disease is to be looked upon as an infection rather than an inheritance; that it is comparatively rarely transmitted from parent to child in utero; adding, however, the opinion that the doctrine of heredity is as yet by no means overthrown. We must still wait for the whole truth.

In the second group of diseases I include those whose bacterial cause has in all probability, but not absolutely, been established. These are leprosy, cholera, typhoid, relapsing fever, pneumonia, diphtheria, gonorrhœa.

It is doubtful whether the leprosy bacilli have ever been successfully cultivated, but transplantation of leprous tissue containing them has repeatedly been followed by a reproduction of the bacilli and the disease. Nor have the spirilla of relapsing fever been obtained by artificial culture. They are, however, always present in the blood in the disease, and successful inoculation is always followed by their appearance in the new victim. The micrococci of gonorrhœa have been artificially cultivated in only a few instances; the procedure is very difficult, and the cultures soon die. A few successful inoculation experiments have been made upon men, but we should like to see a larger measure of proof before we lay aside all doubt. Certain it is, however, that the remaining doubt is very slight.

As to cholera, there is but a shadow of uncertainty remaining that the comma bacilli of Koch are the specific cause of the disease. Whatever uncertainty there is, is due to the lack of inoculation experiments upon man. One accidental case has probably settled the matter, but one case is hardly sufficient. In all other respects the evidence is complete. There has been discovered a rapid method of identifying cholera cultures by the production of a violet-red or purplish-red color upon the addition of pure sulphuric acid. This method may be of great value for the purpose of quick diagnosis in a given case.

The Koch-Eberth typhoid bacillus remains about where it was. It is, in all probability, the specific germ, but in the absence of the final test, i. e., inoculations, some uncertainty remains. Vaughan is skeptical in regard to this bacillus, believing that typhoid may be due to more than one cause; in other words, that it is not a specific disease. Certainly most authorities do not agree with this view.

Of diphtheria, it seems to be about settled that the

bacillus of Loeffler is the specific germ, and that there
is but one cause of genuine diphtheria. The recent
researches of Welch and Abbott in Baltimore have
confirmed this view. It is, however, possible that a
pseudo-membranous disease may be excited by other
agents than the diphtheria bacillus, and Prudden
wisely suggests that it is not best to close the discussion
until all the evidence is in.

As to the germs of pneumonia: The pneumococcus, or pneumo-bacillus, of Friedlander has about lost
its significance. Of it Frænkel says: "Neither microscopic investigation, nor culture, nor transmission
having furnished sufficient proofs for the assertion
that the pneumococci play a decided rôle in the origin
of pneumonia, we cannot recognize them as the causal
factors of this disease." He adds: "It may, therefore, be assumed that they are at any rate related to
the said affection, and it may not be amiss to regard
them (like the streptococci in typhoid) as subsequent
settlers on a soil prepared and properly fitted by the
activity of some other micro-organisms."

The pneumococcus of A. Frænkel, on the other
hand, which, it will be remembered, was first discovered by Sternberg, has risen immensely in importance.
Of it I cannot do better than quote again the words of
Carl Frænkel. "It belongs," he says, "to the most
virulent of infectious micro-organisms known. It is
proved to exist in over 90 per cent. of all cases of
pneumonia. The fact of its being missed here and

there is not difficult to account for, when it is remembered that it cannot be surely recognized by microscopic examination alone, and certain difficulties in its cultivation are not always sufficiently heeded by all observers."

Frænkel's bacteria are by no means exclusively found in pneumonia. They are found in almost all cases of cerebro-spinal meningitis, and the origin of this affection is reasonably attributed to them. A. Frænkel has found them in pleuritis, Weichselbaum in peritonitis, Banti in pericarditis, others have encountered them in endocarditis and otitis media and numerous other affections. They occur especially in the saliva and nasal secretions of healthy persons, as established by Netter, and they may be regarded almost as regular tenants of these localities. Frænkel's diplococcus is indeed not the exciter of pneumonia alone; its domain is more extensive; it does not restrict itself to this one function.

Frænkel's bacterium is perhaps the principal exciter of inflammatory processes of an infectious nature in the human body. Wherever it reaches a serous or mucous membrane and meets with the requirements for its settlement, it commences operations. It causes meningitis on the pia mater, peritonitis on the peritoneum, and otitis in the auditory passage. Whenever it gains entrance into the lungs, pneumonia is developed, the peculiar properties and characteristic procedure of which depend upon the peculiarities of the organ invaded and upon the extent of the morbid process. Another bacterium may eventually play a similar role and give rise to pneumonia, but, as a rule, it is certainly Fraenkel's diplococcus that displays here its energy, for which reason it may properly be regarded as the real micro-organism of genuine croupous lung inflammation.

But how can this view be harmonized with the circumstance that this micro-organism is also a frequent guest in the healthy body; that in the majority of all persons it is domesticated in the mouth, whence it might easily and at all times undertake an excursion into other regions and thus soon produce meningitis, otitis, or something else? Does the "sword of Damocles" actually hang at every moment so close to our heads, and must it not appear almost miraculous that anybody at all is spared by this terrible foe? We can account for this certainly very striking fact only by the circumstance that it requires, as a rule, certain preparatory, as yet unknown, factors to enable this bacterium to make its attacks. The healthy coverings and tissues of the body resist the micro-organisms; only when the native powers of resistance are weakened or neutralized do the foreign invaders take a firm footing and begin their pernicious activity. All the minute gradations of their infectious power (observed even under the conditions of their natural appearance, and surely strong enough to determine the severity of a single case or the character of an epidemic,) will find their explanations in this hypothesis.

Reference ought here to be made to at least one other disease, namely, malaria. It is well known that there has been found a peculiar body in the blood of those suffering from this malady, called after its discoverer the plasmodium of Laveran. It is described as a low organism, not belonging to the class of bacteria, but to the animal kingdom, to be included among the protozoa or mycetozoa, and for this reason named plasmodium. It is found within the red corpuscles. The organism is small, round or irregular, having a rapid amœboid movement; it grows rapidly; soon fills the larger part of the corpuscle, and before long is found to contain many roundish granules or rods consisting of black pigment. It is easily recognized, stained or unstained, in the blood freshly taken from the finger during the attack. It has never been artificially cultivated. Inoculation experiments are therefore wanting. But by agreement among many investigators in Europe and America, it is of great value in diagnosis, enabling us to distinguish with certainty between malaria and other fevers. This fact at once makes it of much practical interest.

Another important matter is now arising in the field of bacteriology. The germ theory of disease is settled; it has become an established fact. But what does it mean and whither is it leading us? Why these

reachings out into such experiments as the Koch
treatment of tuberculosis, the preventive inoculation
against rabies, tetanus and diphtheria? We are approaching the pressing question of immunity, and,
for practical medicine, the greatest problem of our
day: Can we, and how best shall we, combine science
and art to confer upon humanity the inestimable boon
of immunity or cure, or both cure of and immunity
from the infectious diseases?

IV.

SELF-LIMITATION AND IMMUNITY IN DISEASE.

GREAT questions are arising among us as the outgrowth of bacteriology, the most important questions, probably, with which modern medicine has to deal; namely, those concerning self-limitation of and immunity from the infectious diseases. This is the direction in which all eyes are turned, and this is the direction in which we hope to see the triumphs of medicine in the near future. This I say, of course, with the understanding that the broad preventive measures belonging to sanitary science are not under present consideration.

It was not long after the discovery of specific pathogenic bacteria that the question began to be raised: How do these minute organisms produce their effects? Nor was it long before it had been clearly shown that the harm was not done by the mere presence of micro-organisms in the body; in other words, that a mechanical explanation was not sufficient save in a very limited and exceptional way. Almost equally untenable was the theory that the bacteria, in their growth, robbed the body of important substances, to the detriment of the host. Already it had been shown that the new substances arising in the course of the fermentations were the results of the activity of minute living organisms. The yeast is put into the batter; it grows, reproducing itself, spreads through the whole, produces carbonic dioxide and alcohol, and the dough is inflated—made light. Here, then, is proof positive that a small amount of matter may, as the result of its possessing the properties of living things, spread through a large mass, bringing about marked chemical and gross physical changes, the latter being due to the new chemical bodies formed in the process.

So far as the facts were known, the analogy between the fermentations and the infectious diseases was exact. A small quantity of the poison of anthrax being introduced into the body of an animal, or man, in some mysterious way multiplies, spreads through the body, and profoundly modifies it. This poison must be a living thing. Yes, it is proven to be such, and is definitely identified. May not the analogy go further, so that we may say that the modifications are due chiefly to new chemical substances, just as in the fermentations?

That the bacteria do, in the course and as a result of their growth, bring about the formation of new products, and that, in many instances, these are extremely poisonous, is now established, and this knowledge we owe chiefly to the labors of Brieger. The

establishment of this fact at once quickened research
upon the question whether these new products were
not the efficient agents in bringing about the multi-
form and striking effects of infection.

In order to solve the problem, it was necessary to
secure the material for experiments free from living
germs, and for this purpose two processes have been
used, the bacteria under question having been obtained artificially in pure culture. In the first process the cultures were subjected to heat sufficient to
kill the micro-organisms. But it was ascertained that
the heat might also destroy the delicate substances
whose action it was desired to investigate. Recourse
was therefore had to the process of filtration, devised
by Pasteur and Chamberland, and this, or some modification of it, is now generally recognized as the most
reliable method, inasmuch as nothing is destroyed or
changed, the bacteria are removed, and presumably
all of the desired products are secured. Some of
these substances have also been isolated, by definite
chemical processes, from the infected body or from
cultures. Brieger has been the leader in this work,
but thus far it is confessedly difficult, and has yielded
only incomplete results, since bacterial growth is, as a
rule, attended by the formation of several so-called
ptomaines or toxins.

Though the work is beset with difficulties and complications, enough has been established to warrant the
conclusion that the phenomena following infection are

largely, if not entirely, due to the action of new products formed in the growth and multiplication of the
bacteria, and that the peculiar phenomena belonging
to the specific diseases and constituting their specificity
are chiefly, if not wholly, due to the peculiar properties of the ptomaines formed by their specific germs.
Of these phenomena we have now to consider those
two which are of greatest interest to us in our contest
with the infectious diseases, namely, self-limitation
and immunity.

From time immemorial it has been known that
there was a group of diseases which were distinctly
self-limited; they did not run an indefinite course;
they ended of themselves. As the old saying is: "If
the patient lived long enough he would recover from
that disease." To this class of maladies belong
measles, scarlatina, diphtheria, erysipelas, and others.
Here was a great mystery. What was the explanation of it? Theories have been advanced, only to be
disproved or discarded. Those which have not been
disproved have been discarded or held in reserve because there was no way of testing their truth or falsity.

With the rise of modern bacteriology the hope began to be entertained that we might now come nearer
to the solution of the problem. Here again the analogy between the fermentations and the infectious diseases threw a light along the way, indicating the direction for the investigation to proceed. It is known
of certain fermentations not only that they are accom-

panied by the formation of new chemical bodies, but
that through the agency of these substances the fermentation is stopped. In a word, the process is self-
limiting; the ferment is drowned, or benumbed, in its
own products. Some of these bodies are known; they
are recognizable by ordinary chemical methods, and
by their use we may imitate, artificially and exactly,
the natural self-limitation of the processes by which
they are produced. All this is true of the ordinary
alcoholic fermentation.

Of course, the question arose whether something of
the same kind might not explain the phenomena of
the self-limited diseases. Might it not be that the
new compounds resulting from the growth of the
germs in the body, either by altering the soil on which
they grow or actually poisoning them, bring the disease to an end, and thus be explained one of the greatest direct life-saving agencies known to man? Certainly the analogy from the fermentation would seem
to warrant the inference which experiments, so far
made, tend only to confirm. It might be said that
the apparent self-limitation is no real self-limitation,
but only a subsidence of the disease accompanying the
completion of the cycle of the germ's natural life-
history. But such an explanation is untenable, for
there is no such cycle of life-history in the sense just
indicated. Given the proper conditions and suitable
food, and the germs will continue to multiply and reproduce themselves indefinitely. Nor is the theory

of the exhaustion of the available food-supply any more tenable. It is sufficiently disproved by the fact that in some diseases, which are distinctly self-limited, as tetanus, diphtheria and erysipelas, the germ growth is confined to a small spot in the body. And yet in case of diseases in which one attack does not afford protection against others, the same germs may, soon after the first attack, be successfully implanted in another part of the body, and the same phenomena of self-limitation of the disease be seen. The proper food is evidently not exhausted.

Why do not the germs continue to grow indefinitely in the body? Why do they die out with such regularity? Apparently but one explanation remains. There must be some actual interference with their further growth, either in a temporary or permanent modification of the tissues, which renders them unfit for the sustenance of that special germ, or in an agent which directly antagonizes or even kills it. This is the belief which is now generally and with good reason entertained, and upon it are based the most active and perhaps most promising efforts to attack the cause of the infectious diseases even after they have invaded the body.

But there is another fact, long known, concerning certain of the infectious diseases, equally astonishing and life-saving as self-limitation, namely, self-protection, or immunity. It is true of some of these maladies that one attack protects against others; the body, if haply it survives the first, is endowed with an immunity from subsequent infection by the same germ.

Here is a phenomenon quite different from self-limitation, and requiring, perhaps, a different explanation, for they are by no means commensurate, nor even co-existent in the history of a disease. The one may be present, the other absent; one may be strongly marked, the other moderate, or but very slight. Apparently, therefore, they do not necessarily depend upon one or the same cause; indeed, there is reason to believe that, in some diseases, at least, they result from quite different causes, and are brought about in different ways.

Can we explain immunity, or, if not, can we discover and imitate the process by which it is established? Here, too, theory has run riot in the field where knowledge was wanting, but a satisfactory conclusion has not yet been reached. Of these theories the following are worthy of mention: First, that of exhaustion; that the growth of the germs exhausts the nutritive substances necessary for their life, thus leaving the body incapable of supporting the germs in the future. This explanation is now believed to be untenable, for reasons previously stated. Second, the theory of retention; that some peculiar substance is left in the body which antagonizes the germs should they subsequently enter. Of this Frænkel says it is possible, though not probable, and may be retained as a working hypothesis. Third, the phagocytosis the-

4

ory of Metschnikoff, which explains immunity thus:
that the cells, especially the leucocytes, have conferred
upon them, as the result of the first attack, the special
property of subsequently devouring and destroying
the same germs.   Fourth, the theory of the germicidal power of the blood serum.   It is known that
certain animals are naturally unsusceptible to certain
diseases, and that the introduction of their blood serum into susceptible animals may confer upon them a
more or less lasting power of resisting those germs to
which the first animal was naturally immune.   This
is the theory upon which was based the goat blood and
dog blood treatment of tuberculosis.

Of these theories Fraenkel observes that there is
probably a truth in all, and that artificial immunity is
not acquired by one regular process, but sometimes in
this manner, sometimes in that, and that it is quite
possible and even probable that causes are at-work
which are as yet unknown, and which future investigators are destined to discover.   But whatever the
manner of action, the primary fact remains that in
certain diseases the growth of the germs in the body
leaves it protected against a subsequent invasion of
the same germ; and further, that this acquired immunity is brought about through the agency of the
new chemical bodies evolved during the germ growth.

Naturally, the knowledge of these facts has given
rise to an extensive series of experiments, all having
for their object the imitation of nature in securing

immunity. This work has not been without striking results. There are several diseases, such as anthrax, symptomatic anthrax, swine erysipelas, and, perhaps, tetanus, rabies and diphtheria, the attack upon which has shown an encouraging degree of success.

It will be seen that, as a practical matter, the imitation of natural self-limitation and immunity, that is, cutting short or curing, and protecting against infection, present quite different problems.

Here rises into prominence another matter. As already stated, bacterial growth is often or usually accompanied by the formation of several new compounds. Which of these is the effective agent in the self-limitation, and which in affording immunity? Are the substances which do the harm and render the disease dangerous the same as those which do the good? This is a question of great importance, especially when we come to the problem of imitating self-limitation and thereby cutting short and curing a disease. If the harmful and helpful agents are the same, it is open to question whether we may legitimately introduce into a body already suffering under an active disease an agent which, while re-enforcing the tendency to self-cure, may also increase the tendency to death. Under these conditions it would seem that such treatment could, at best, be of value only in the earliest stage of the disease, and in this way only was it that Koch hoped to do good by the use of his "lymph" against tuberculosis. If the harmful and helpful

agents are different, then, could we but isolate the
latter, we might use it at any stage of the disease, and
only with benefit.

Then, too, the question arises whether the agents
producing self-limitation and immunity are the same,
and the possibility, if different, of separating and obtaining them for practical use. We must also ask
ourselves whether it is always or usually possible to
obtain the desired substances from artificial cultures
of the germs. May there not be processes attending
the growth of the germs in the living body which are
not possible in the artificial experiments? For, as
Fraenkel aptly reminds us, the living tissue is no plate
of gelatine and no test-tube. How far this may prove
an obstacle to progress is as yet uncertain; but it is
certain that it does not necessarily and always forbid
success by the artificial method.

Here we see two schools of experimenters arising.
The one excludes the living germ, seeking and using
only the sterile germ products. This they do under
the belief that, could the problems indicated be solved,
and the processes be worked out to exactness by chemistry, the method would be more accurate and less
dangerous. For, thus far, experiments made with
even weakened living germs have proven to be accompanied by more or less risk.

The other school, acting upon the conviction that
artificial culture cannot be relied upon to produce the
same results as germ-growth in the living tissues, uses

the living germs, but weakened, claiming thus to more closely imitate nature. This weakening or attenuation of the virus is brought about in various ways: by altering the culture soil, by heat, gases, varying atmospheric pressure, drying, and by passing the germs through the bodies of animals. Pasteur started the line of work which has made him famous upon the supposition that vaccinia was simply smallpox modified by passing through the body of the cow. Whether this is true or not, his theory of the use of attenuated virus proved correct, and led to the astonishing results in the diseases already mentioned. Which line of work will best sustain its claims in the end remains for the future to decide. Certainly thus far the living virus seems to have the more to its credit.

Let us now look for a moment at several other interesting facts, to which I shall refer but briefly before attempting to sum up the matter of our discussion.

First, as already indicated, the blood, or body juices, of animals, naturally immune, may afford more or less protection to susceptible animals against a disease to which the one is immune. This fact may open the way to some valuable results.

Second, it may ultimately be found that the apparent absence, or slight tendency to self-limitation and immunity in certain diseases, is only apparent; that these tendencies are present, but are overcome by an-

tagonizing agents. If, then, it shall be found that
the harmful and the helpful agents are different, and
the latter can be separately obtained, we may be able
to use them successfully even in diseases, such as tuberculosis, which, under ordinary conditions, show
little or no tendency to self-limitation or immunity.
Such an effort has been made with the tuberculin of
Koch.

Third, It has long been observed that the presence
of certain diseases in the body seemed to exclude, or
oppose, the entrance of others, and it is now known
that there is an antagonism between certain bacteria.
Such antagonism may be shown, not only on the cul-
ture-plate, but in the body. Thus, rabbits inoculated
with the intensely virulent anthrax may be saved from
death by introducing, shortly before or after such
inoculation, the micrococcus prodigiosus. Here is an
example of cure of a malignant disease: If cowpox
is not simply modified smallpox, vaccination may be
said to be an example of immunity afforded through
such antagonism. In both examples the beneficial
agent is practically harmless. It is by no means impossible that here may be found a clue to success with
our efforts.

In conclusion, let us sum up the whole matter and
see where we stand to-day, and what grounds we have
for entertaining a hopeful prospect. It will be no-
ticed, as we review the questions under discussion and
study the various plans suggested by bacteriological

investigations for the attack upon the infectious diseases, that they fall into two general groups: First, those based upon the facts observed in the ordinary course of the infectious diseases; second, those based upon facts coming from other directions. What expectation or hopes open now before us in this great field?

If, as to the questions of self-limitation and immunity, we study the infectious diseases, we shall find that they fall into three quite distinct classes.

First, there is a class of these diseases in which both self-limitation and immunity are practically absolute. Such are measles, scarlatina, smallpox, typhoid fever. This being true, we might hope to command the situation, so far as immunity is concerned, if we could secure an attenuated virus or the chemical products of their germs. It would hardly seem that we could expect to accomplish much in the way of cure, even by an attenuated virus, since by this process we should subject the already crippled body to something of the harmful as well as helpful agents. But provided these agents are different, and we could obtain the latter, we might then have settled even the matter of cure.

The second class includes diseases in which self-limitation is absolute, but subsequent immunity is slight, or wanting. Here we find such affections as diphtheria, erysipelas and pneumonia. With these the problem of cure would be the same as before. But what of immunity? If the natural process does not afford it, experiment along this line would not seem promising.

Of the third class, in which both self-limitation and immunity are slight or wanting, tuberculosis is a type. And here the prospect in either direction seems dark. With the facts of the natural history before us, what can be expected from an imitation of that process? And yet the suggestion hitherto made in regard to tuberculosis may be true. It may be that there is an agent of self-limitation which only waits to be found and isolated, which, freed from the antagonism of others, may furnish an unexpected escape from defeat. Or here, and elsewhere, where the outlook seems very doubtful, the facts coming in other directions may give light, indicating that the way to success is to be sought, not in initiating the natural course of events, but in utilizing agents obtained from animals possessing a natural immunity; by pushing further the investigations upon the antagonism between different bacteria, or by some means yet to be discovered. If it is possible to cure malaria by quinine; to drown the yeast germ in its own secretion; to guard against diphtheria or tetanus by the blood of protected animals; to jugulate malignant anthrax by the harmless prodigiosus, why should it be thought impossible to carry the work farther, to conquer even the great destroyer, tuberculosis?

The contest is really but just begun, and we are, as

yet, too often at the mercy of the almost invisible foes which prey upon and destroy the majority of our race. But we are steadily advancing in knowledge, which is power, and one day we shall conquer. It may be by this means, it may be by that, but we shall conquer. One day, we believe, we shall issue to the pestiferous brood the authoritative command: Out upon you; hence, begone!

V.

THE CONTEST AGAINST INFECTION.

IT has become evident that bacteriology is now progressing chiefly in the direction of discovering the channels through which the self-limitation of and immunity from infectious diseases is brought about. As stated heretofore, enough has been learned to establish the principle that the effects of bacteria are produced by chemical substances contained in their bodies or resulting from the growth of these bacteria. Sufficient also has been learned to show that self-limitation and immunity are in some way the outcome of such substances. The question, therefore, presents itself: What is immunity, and through what channels and by what agents is it brought about?

At the outset we must recognize two forms of immunity: first, natural immunity, by which is meant a natural insusceptibility of certain animals to certain diseases; second, acquired immunity.

Acquired immunity may be brought about in three ways: First, by an attack of the disease; second, by inoculation with an allied disease or with the disease modified by passing the virus through another animal;

third, by the virus modified by culture outside of the body. How are these results brought about?

Among the various theories are two which have assumed prominence. First, the phagocytosis theory of Metschnikoff, which supposes that certain cells of the body are active agents in the warfare against infection. In following out this theory Metschnikoff has displayed a remarkable degree of ingenuity, patience and skill, and has brought out some exceedingly interesting and important facts. The other theory is that the protective agents are to be found in the blood and body juices. As the result of the work of the last year or two it must be said that opinion tends strongly in the direction of the second view. Von Fodor finds, as the result of a series of experiments and researches, that arterial blood has more anti-bacterial influence than venous; that fresh blood has more influence than old; that the maximum anti-bacterial power of the blood is at the temperature of 100° to 104° F.; that the individual susceptibility of an animal to an infectious disease seems to be in direct relationship to the germicidal power of its blood; that various chemical and other agents diminish while others increase this power, the most marked increase being brought about by carbonate of sodium and potassium. He concluded that any agent which increases the alkalinity of the blood increased the resisting power of the organism against bacteria. A series of experiments made on this basis seems to prove the correctness of the theory.

60 ESSAYS ON BACTERIOLOGY.

Naturally, as the result of these discoveries, the attempt has been made to find a bactericidal agent in the blood. Hankin has been a leader in this special work. He believes that he has established, for certain animals at least, that the blood contains a substance of a proteid nature which belongs to the globulins and has certain bactericidal properties. Following this supposition, he was able to neutralize inoculations of anthrax by injection of a solution of this globulin. The tendency of investigation is unmistakably in at least the general direction of Hankin's view.

These albuminoid substances have been called defensive proteids, and investigation seems to indicate that they may act in one of three ways: first, by killing the bacteria, that is, microbicidal; second, by attenuating or weakening the bacteria; third, by neutralizing or destroying the toxines. In justice to the work of Metschnikoff it must be said that this blood serum theory does not necessarily disprove his phagocytosis theory, for it is still quite possible that self-limitation or immunity, or both, may result from these defensive proteids acting upon or through the cells.

Behring and Kitasato found that the serum of rabbits vaccinated against tetanus had the property of destroying the toxin of tetanus in guinea pigs, so that guinea pigs might be cured of tetanus by injection of rabbit serum taken from vaccinated rabbits. The same authors proved a similar fact in regard to diphthoria. Already it is reported that clinical use has been made of this discovery in actually curing some six or seven cases of tetanus in men. The first experiments in this direction were made by transfusion of the whole blood. Subsequently it was found that the protecting properties resided not in the corpuscles but in the serum.

It is to be noted here that these defensive proteids are not general in their action; that is, serum, or a defensive proteid derived from it, which will protect against one disease will not necessarily protect against others. We cannot, therefore, at present entertain the idea of discovering a universal bactericidal agent of blood serum, sufficient at least for use as a general protective. Hankin suggests a classification of these defensive proteids into two groups: first, those existing naturally in animals, and these he calls sozins; second, those existing in animals artificially made immune, which he calls phyloxins. For sub-classes he suggests the prefixes mico- and toxo- to indicate sozins or phyloxins which destroy bacteria or which destroy toxins. Emmerich, in summing up his researches, claims to have established two important principles: first, that the cause of artificial immunity is an anti-bacterial substance which is not injurious to the body; and second, that the protective fluid for one class of animals may be applied against that particular disease in other classes of animals. For instance, that the fluid from protected rabbits could be successfully used to cure infected swine. He claims, says Ernst, that he has by these experiments entered upon the first stage of a certain and rational treatment of infectious disease, and urges it to be the duty of all to strive for the attainment of an ideal that must complete the discovery and manufacture of the true anti-bacterial material. The time is perhaps not far distant when such a material will be in the hands of all who are called on to treat infectious diseases. Other diseases besides swine fever are already under investigation. It will be noted by the study of this whole matter that the tendency now is to use the natural laboratory, that is, the living body, rather than artificial cultures to secure those protective agents.

In summing up this matter, in order to indicate the present status of the contest against infection, I make the following brief statement as an indication of the best present opinion:

First. The infectious diseases are due to living agents.

Second. Bacteria injure the body and cause sickness through the production of poisonous substances called, loosely, ptomaines or toxins.

Third. Self-limitation and immunity are in some way, directly or indirectly, brought about by the action of such chemical substances, the protective agents, however, not being necessarily the same as those which cause the sickness.

Fourth. These protective agents may be found in the blood serum and body juices.

Fifth. Their protective action may be a direct one, or it may be exerted through certain cells called phagocytes, the former seeming at present the most probable.

Sixth. Natural or acquired immunity may be transferred from one animal to another by the transfer of blood serum.

Seventh. Following out the indications from these facts, sufficient practical success has been achieved to make the most conservative almost an enthusiast, and to furnish ground for a rational hope and expectation of further success.

The following prediction is made by Ernst: "In spite of the great number of unknown points that still surround this new theory of immunity by defensive proteids, it can already be predicted that it will come out victorious in the struggle in which it is engaged, with the numberless hypotheses and the old prejudices that surround and encumber this branch of general pathology. It will be victorious, for it has already given certain proofs of its importance by vaccinating and curing animals by means of these defensive proteids."

A brief review now of work done with some of the specific bacteria:

1. Cholera.—Nothing has really been done to overthrow Koch's previous work. Klein, of London, has expressed skepticism in regard to the comma bacillus of cholera as a specific organism, quoting the in-

vestigations of Cunningham, in India, who claims to
have recognized several different species of comma
bacilli in cholera. The value and meaning of these
claims remain as yet doubtful. It is interesting to
note the experiment of Pettenkofer, who voluntarily
swallowed pure cultures of comma bacilli brought
fresh from Hamburg. He did this to show his con-
tempt for these organisms as the active cause of cholera. The result of his self-inoculation was a moderate sickness, which he asserted not to be cholera, but
which less prejudiced authorities believe to have been
simply a mild cholera, the discharges from the bowels
containing almost pure cultures of the comma bacilli.
Another experimenter, actuated by the same motive,
produced in himself similar results, except that the
sickness was more severe. It is of practical interest
also that, upon the approach of cholera to New York
recently, the presence of the comma bacilli in the de-
jections was successfully used as a test of the existence of the disease in suspected cases.

2. Cancer.—Many observations have been made
of peculiar bodies in cancerous tissue. These have
mostly been placed in the class coccidia. Their investigation is so difficult, artificial cultivation so elu-
sive, and their relation to the tissue cells so peculiar,
that it is difficult to decide their biological position.
The question is, therefore, still unsettled. Domergue
is inclined to believe these coccidia to be simply cell
transformations. There are, however, those who take
a different view, who believe them to be true parasites.

3. Dysentery.—Evidence upon the pathogenic properties of the amœba coli has been accumulating. Kartulis claims to have secured pure cultures of the amœba in decoctions of fresh straw. He claims also to have made successful inoculations in cats. Owing to the work of many foreign investigators and of Councilman, Welsh, Osler and others in America, the diagnostic value of the amœba coli seems to have been well established, as also its causative relation to other than dysenteric lesions, especially to hepatic abscesses.

4. Diphtheria.—No important change has occurred in the bacteriology of this disease. Previous opinions have simply been strengthened. Recent investigations seem to show that the diphtheria bacilli are secondarily diffused through the body more frequently than has been heretofore supposed. The most important work on diphtheria has been that already mentioned, namely, the successful protective and curative experiments of Behring and Kitasato.

5. Erysipelas.—The uncertainty as to the identity of the streptococcus of erysipelas and the streptococcus pyogenes remains. Fraenkel, among others, has done work which seems to give additional proof of the identity of these organisms.

6. Gonorrhœa.—I have only to repeat and emphasize a statement made in a former report, that while the microscopic discovery of the gonococcus may be looked upon as very strong evidence for pathological and clinical purposes, its medico-legal value is

5

doubtful. We are not in position as yet to make absolute statements in court as to the diagnostic importance of the gonococcus, at least as found by the microscope alone.

7. Smallpox and Vaccination.—Renewed interest has been taken and renewed activity shown in investigating the question of the identity of variola and vaccinia. Unmistakably the tendency of experiments is to confirm the view that vaccinia is nothing but variola modified by passing through the cow. This might and would seem strange were it not for the fact that the last ten years has shown that the virus of many other diseases may be much modified by passage through the body of certain animals. It is quite possible that we shall soon have established the fact that variola is inoculable upon the cow, if the inoculation is properly made—that such inoculation becomes changed after efficient repetition into vaccinia, and that inoculation in this way affords an always controllable means of obtaining animal vaccine.

8. Bacillus Pyocyaneus.—The microbe of green pus has risen into prominence and importance, chiefly because of its remarkable influence in arresting the development of anthrax when inoculated at about the same time as that virulent germ.

9. Malaria.—The diagnostic value of the malarial plasmodia remains high; indeed, the best opinion tends to make it absolute. The work of Osler, Welsh, and Councilman in this country, and of Laveran,

Golgi, Rosenbach and others among foreigners, has continued. Rosenbach has shown the interesting fact that the malarial parasite can be kept alive for at least forty-eight hours in the digestive canal of the leech.

10. Purulent Pleurisy.—The subject of purulent pleurisy has continued to attract investigation. The result is a tendency to include all, or nearly all, purulent plurisies in three groups: First, those due to the Sternberg-Frenkel pneumococcus; second, those excited by the pyogenic staphylococci; third, those due to tubercle bacilli. Microscopic examination or cultivation or inoculation experiments will show the character of the case; and of this knowledge real, practical clinical use may be made.

11. Tetanus.—The previously expressed views as to the specific nature of the tetanus bacilli have been confirmed. Every one now believes that the specific bacterial origin of this disease has been established. The most interesting outcome of recent work has been the prevention and cure of tetanus by the use of blood serum or defensive proteids. Mention has already been made of the apparently successful practice of such cure upon men.

12. Tuberculosis.—Time only increases our admiration of the marvelous piece of scientific work revealed in Koch's announcement of his discovery of the specific cause of tuberculosis. Time also only adds emphasis to the practical diagnostic value of this dis-

covery and the importance of its daily use. Some improvements have been made in the methods of examining sputum which enable us to reach certainty in otherwise doubtful cases. These are, first, liquefaction of the sputum by the addition of a small quantity of dilute sodium hydrate. Such liquefied sputum is allowed to settle in a conical vessel, and the sediment examined for bacilli by the ordinary means. Second, the addition of liquid carbolic acid precipitates the bacilli-containing masses in the sputum, which may be examined with increased prospect of finding the few bacilli present. Third, the centrifugal machine has been applied for a similar purpose, just as it is applied to secure the rapid deposits of urinary casts.

I would, in this connection, emphasize the value and simplicity of inoculations upon rabbits or guinea pigs for diagnostic purposes in otherwise obscure cases.

So far as we can now tell, the tuberculin experiment of Koch to arrest tuberculosis has been a failure. We now know more of the reason for expecting such failure than we did when the treatment was promulgated. However, no one conversant with the progress of bacteriology supposes for a moment that this failure will, or should, dishearten us or arrest further experiment in this and other diseases. Through the work of Hunter, Cheyne, Klebs and others it has been shown that even Koch himself was ignorant of the substance with which he was dealing, the two former authors having thought to modify and improve Koch's tuberculin by excluding some of the harmful constituents. Klebs has claimed to accomplish the same result, and considerable interest has been taken in his modified tuberculin, the so-called tuberculo-cidin. In spite of these claims, it is evident that the results gained by following this particular line of experiments has not been great. It evidently yet remains to find an agent which approaches a specific for tuberculosis. Nevertheless, bearing in mind the remarkable developments of the last few years, the great progress made in clearing up the mystery of proteids, and remembering the astonishing antagonism which may exist between different bacteria, even between harmless and virulent ones, there is certainly room for hope. I believe that the day will come, it may come soon, it may be long delayed, but the day will come when tuberculosis will be as thoroughly at our mercy as is smallpox to-day. It will have sunk to the insignificance of a beaten and imprisoned enemy. I hope and expect to see it before my hair has grown gray.

VI

RETROSPECT AND PROSPECT OF PROGRESS.

FOUR years have passed since the paper upon "Some Problems of Bacteriology" was written. Times change and we change with them, and such change is no disgrace provided it consists in progress toward truth. That during these four years modifications of views have come about, supposed facts have been shown to be deceptive, new truths have come to light and broader conceptions of matters bacteriological have developed, goes without saying.

It may, therefore, not be out of place to review some of the statements contained in former essays, that we may see how far modifications are necessary to adapt these statements to present knowledge, and how much nearer we have come to established truth. As we proceed in this review it will become evident that in some directions there has been a simplification which is to be expected as the field clears and we come nearer to the great and fundamental truths.

In other directions progress has served but to show into what an immense field we have entered. In some directions final truth has been reached or is near at hand; in others it is evidently as yet afar off. But the prospect is inviting; progress brings a constant succession of fulfilled expectations, equally unexpected disappointments, startling surprises, suddenly opening avenues for the advance, and that the final results will be great and good no one can doubt.

We are still confronted by the difficulty in making satisfactory inoculation tests in several of the important diseases, the specific bacteria of which are all but demonstrated. This is still true of typhoid fever and Asiatic cholera. So far as we know, animals are not subject to these diseases, at least not in a definitely recognizable form. While, therefore, there can be little doubt that the Koch-Eberth bacillus and the Koch spirillum are the genuine exciters of these diseases, the final and absolute step in the demonstration remains to be taken. Several bold experimenters have swallowed fresh cultures of cholera spirilla, in several instances inducing moderate attacks of a disorder similar to cholera, with swarms of the organisms in the stools. Among these daring men was the veteran Pettenkofer, whose object was to show that other factors than the germs were at least active in the production of the disease. In one instance, under the observation of the well-known Metschnikoff, a man in Paris induced a typical attack of cholera by swallowing a pure culture, and that in the absence of cholera in Paris at the time. This is held by some to be conclusive evidence; but we can hardly be satisfied without a more thorough test.

Even though this obstacle to experiment remain, there are other, though indirect, means of demonstrating the specific relation of a given bacterium to a disease. For instance, if it be shown that a certain germ may be used to furnish a successful vaccine, a defensive proteid, or immunizing blood serum, against the disease from which it was obtained, the fact goes far toward proving that germ to be the specific exciter of that disease. Thus the road, blocked in one direction, opens up in another.

As to the question whether each of the infectious diseases has a single specific causative agent, the answer may now be more satisfactory. There are some maladies of which it seems to have been abundantly shown that this is true; for instance, tuberculosis and glanders. There are others, however, which have ordinarily been looked upon as specific diseases, of which we now take a different view. Among these are the septic and inflammatory affections "which do not present such sharp and definite differential characters as do those more specific infectious diseases which are caused by only a single species of micro-organism. Some of these present clinical and pathological differences in accordance with their etiological differences, whereas others do not. To this class belong acute ulcerative endocarditis, meningitis, broncho-pneumonia, erysipelas, pyemia, septicemia, osteomyelitis, and puerperal fever. Most of these names are simply collective terms for different diseases which have already received, or are likely still further to receive, more exact definition as the result of bacteriological studies." (Welch).

Upon antisepsis and disinfection there is little new to be said. They have been worked out, for all practical purposes, to fair satisfaction. The methods of testing disinfectants remain as before; their practical application is being constantly improved, but in details only. Every one knows that asepsis in surgery has taken precedence over antisepsis as formerly applied, and every one understands the reasons for the change. The reason is simply the old one that prevention is better than cure. But, be it remembered, there is still and there will doubtless remain an important field for antisepsis, and for just the same reasons that there remains and will remain the necessity for curative as well as preventive measures in general medical practice. The necessity for antisepsis and for curative measures will remain just as long as infecting and other pathogenic agents precede the advent of the surgeon or physician.

Investigators are still battling with the problem of the hereditary transmission of the infectious diseases, and the matter is by no means yet settled.

It is settled that offspring may come into the world with the germs of disease in their bodies. But just how frequent this is and how far it must be taken into account in everyday practice and sanitary science, is, with some diseases, still uncertain. Here, as always, interest centers around tuberculosis. It is generally conceded that family history plays an important role in this disease; but whether this is to be laid chiefly to the charge of some general or special predisposition, of infection growing out of closer association or of house contamination, or of actual hereditary transmission of the disease germs, remains open to debate. Baumgarten has steadfastly and earnestly advocated the latter view, which is rendered more plausible by the accumulating facts as to the possibility of tubercle germs remaining long latent in the living body. Yet there are many things to be explained before we can accept Baumgarten's view. In the meantime nothing has been brought to light to in any way shake the great truth that tuberculosis is to be included among the specific infectious diseases, and that multitudes are falling victims to this infection in the ordinary way. The chronic character of the malady, the many secondary factors influencing its inception and progress, and above all its long period of incubation, these things alone prevent the general recognition of its infectious character as clearly as that of measles, scarlatina or smallpox. Surely the time will not be long before failure of such recognition and consequent action will be properly held as evidence of criminal neglect.

In a former paper I endeavored to summarize briefly the status of our knowledge as to the relationship between particular disease and particular bac-

teria. Something additional may be acceptable in
this line to bring the subject up to date.

First, Tuberculosis.—One of the most important
matters in the study of this disease has been the demonstration that tubercle bacilli may long remain latent
or dormant in the body, to be called into activity by
various exciting agencies. Thus the bronchial glands
have been repeatedly shown to contain living tubercle
bacilli while the lungs and other organs were apparently free both from the germs and the disease. This
fact doubtless explains many cases of acute tuberculosis following such diseases as measles, whooping
cough and typhoid fever, and slight wounds to bones
and joints. Furthermore, proof positive has been accumulating that actual congenital transmission of tuberculosis is more frequent than was a few years ago
supposed. To be sure, these demonstrations have
been comparatively few, but they seem to strengthen
the view of Baumgarten, to which reference has already been made.

A review of tuberculosis would be incomplete without reference to the efforts which are being awakened
the world over to limit the spread of the disease by
limiting the distribution of the poison. Already a
number of foreign and American sanitary boards have
instituted formal measures in this direction. The
New York City Board of Health has here again demonstrated its progressive efficiency. The question of
compulsory notification of tuberculosis has given rise

to sharp debate, for well-known reasons; but upon the necessity of some measures to restrict the reckless spread of this dread agent of destruction, there can be no difference of opinion. The fact that the material coming from tuberculous lesions contains a living poison, capable, whether upon the clothing, the floors, the walls, or in the dust of the air, of exciting the disease; this fact, I say, is sufficient warrant for some measures looking to the protection of the public against the danger. But whatever is done must be done carefully, wisely, and under the direction of those who understand the facts and the conditions under which the action must be carried out, and who can take broad, well-balanced views of the situation.

Tetanus.—There seems to be no longer any question that the tetanus bacillus of Nicolaier and Kitasato is the specific cause of that malady. This has been confirmed not only by the cultivation and inoculation experiments, but in the production of artificial immunity through the agency of the same germ. Reference will be made to this matter later.

Diphtheria.—There is now an apparently unanimous opinion that the Klebs-Loeffler bacillus is the specific cause of diphtheria; that the exudative sore throats accompanying scarlatina, measles, and other acute diseases, while sometimes diphtheria, are usually of different origin, though not rarely of no less gravity. It seems further agreed that the examination for the Klebs-Loeffler bacillus may be made of

great practical value in diagnosis. Further, it has
been shown that, while the diphtheria bacilli are not
usually disseminated through the body, they may be
carried about and set up secondary infection, giving
rise to acute ulcerative endocarditis and other lesions.
Finally, we are apparently nearing a solution of the
vexed question of the relationship between diphtheria
and membranous croup. The writer has reported some
investigations in this line. Of late several boards of
health, which are conducted upon scientific rather
than political lines, have been giving close study to
the problem, and with somewhat startling results.
The pathologists of the New York board have examined several hundred reported cases of membranous
croup, finding the diphtheria germs present in about
80 per cent. Corresponding results have been
reached in other cities. The New York board has
therefore recommended that membranous croup, so
called, should be included among the diseases to be
reported by the physician for the purpose of institut-
ing protective measures. Whether all cases of membranous croup are simply laryngeal diphtheria remains to be settled by further and more exhaustive
studies. In the meantime it may fairly be asked
whether the report of about a hundred deaths from
membranous croup in this city during the last three
years does not come near to being an example of gross
professional carelessness.

Something more might be said in regard to some of

the specific bacteria, but perhaps little of importance in addition to what has already been said. I turn, therefore, to a brief survey of that rising field of work in which all are deeply interested, namely, the investigations upon immunity from and protection against the infectious diseases.

An immense amount of work is being done in this direction; hap-hazard experiments are becoming fewer, and the whole matter is steadily being reduced to a more scientific basis. We now recognize several ways of securing a more or less lasting immunity against many of these diseases, and there is opening up a new field, already promising, in the way of cure for those laboring under an attack. It would require a long time to even briefly review this great mass of work, and present its results. I can, therefore, only note some interesting and leading points. As I have said, there are several ways by which a more or less lasting immunity may be secured.

First. By inoculation of such amounts of living and virulent cultures of the microbe causing the disease as shall fall short of a fatal result. An example of this was the practice of inoculation against small-pox, which preceded the far safer and about as equally successful vaccination worked out by Jenner.

Second. Inoculation of the specific microbe partly or wholly attenuated in virulence, this attenuation being secured by various means, such as culture under peculiar conditions, or passing the germs through the bodies of certain animals. Of this method the vaccination of Jenner is probably an example.

Third. The injection of products of the specific bacteria, these products being obtained from cultures or from the bodies of infected animals. They may be used when still toxic, or, more frequently, after diminution or removal of their toxicity.

The principal means of reducing toxicity and increasing vaccinating values are heat and mixture with certain animal juices, particularly thymus extract, or with tri-chloride of iodine and some other agents injurious to bacterial poisons.

The so-called chemical vaccines belong to this class. They have a very wide field of application. In some instances partial immunity has followed the introduction of this class of substances into the stomach.

Fourth. Injection of blood-serum or other fluids from animals artificially rendered immune from the disease. As the blood-serum from immunized animals may possess not only prophylactic but curative properties, it has been called curative or healing serum.

Usually various methods can be successfully employed in producing artificial immunity from a given disease.

It is a general rule that a given microbe and its products are capable of conferring immunity only from the disease which is caused by that microbe.

The conferred immunity may be increased in degree and durability by the gradual use of vaccines of increasing strength, followed by inoculations of the virulent microbes or their products, until an astonishingly high degree of insusceptibility may be reached; such a degree, indeed, that immense quantities of the most virulent microbes may be introduced without harm.

Following some of these methods of immunization, an animal may sometimes be protected against the growth of the bacteria in the body, while it still remains susceptible to the toxic products of that bacterium; and vice versa.

Some of the so-called antitoxins obtained from the blood serum may be obtained in far greater concentration than that in which they exist in the original fluids. It is to be hoped that this work may be carried still further.

It has been found that, once an animal has been successfully immunized, the successive injection of increasing quantities of the toxic substances may bring about an enormous increase in the antitoxic or immunizing power of the body fluid of that animal. In tetanus, for instance, the point may thus be reached where 1 c. c. of serum is sufficient to immunize 500,000 mice weighing 20 grm. each, or 200 sheep of ordinary weight.

The blood-serum therapy for the cure of disease already under way has been most thoroughly worked out in diphtheria and tetanus. The curative value of the serum is in direct proportion to the quantity introduced and to the degree of immunity previously conferred upon the animal from which the serum was obtained.

The stage and intensity of the attack have much influence upon the results obtained by this blood-serum therapy. The longer the attack has lasted and the more intense it is, the greater the quantity of serum necessary to arrest its progress. This resistance to the serum rises very rapidly, so rapidly, indeed, as to soon reach such a point as to require an amount of serum impossible to introduce into the animal. Hence the desirability of progress in the direction of securing the immunizing or curative agent from the serum in some more concentrated form. In regard to the difficulty just referred to, it is less in diphtheria than in tetanus.

There are still many difficulties in the application of this serum therapy to the larger animals and to man. Already considerable success seems to have been reached in its application to human tetanus and diphtheria, but it is yet too early to predict what the outcome may be. The conditions in the laboratory are quite different from those at the bedside, and we must be careful how we carry over inferences and experiments from one to the other. At present we can but maintain an attitude of hopeful expectation, strong in the conviction that sooner or later every gain in knowledge will result in practical good.

6

VII.

ANTITOXIC SERUM THERAPY.

IN view of recent events, the consideration of serum therapy in general and of the antitoxic serum treatment of diphtheria in particular is of the greatest interest. Reference has been made to the progress of investigations in this direction, and to the fact that already this new principle of treatment, prophylactic and curative, had been brought to the point of a practical test. As every one knows, it has engaged the intense interest and attention of the world. Having thus established for itself a place in the history of medical progress, it will be well to briefly survey its origin and development.

I have already discussed the various methods, the outgrowths of modern bacteriology, which have, with more or less success, been tried in the attempt to imitate or improve upon nature in securing an immunity from or cure of infectious diseases. These experiments have been based upon the discovery that, the infectious diseases being due to germs, their phenomena, including self-cure, and subsequent immunity, were in some way the results of the presence of the chemical products of germs acting upon the living organism. In the endeavor to imitate or improve upon nature in this direction the tendency has been unmistakably to make use of what may be called the natural laboratory, that is, the animal body.

Several important discoveries have combined to give us the new serum therapy.

1. It was found that the blood and other body fluids had a certain amount of bactericidal power. This may be said to have been the starting point of the long line of investigations which have centered in the blood.

2. It was found that, imitating nature, animals could be rendered immune to certain diseases by introducing into their bodies the germs or the toxic products of the specific germs which caused the diseases.

3. Carrying these experiments further, it was found that by a process of progressive inoculations from weaker to more virulent germs, or of injections of smaller to larger quantities of toxins, a progressive degree of resisting power to those germs or toxins could be developed. The degree to which this rise of resisting power can be carried is indeed astonishing.

4. When the agency of this artificially induced resisting power came to be investigated, it was found to apparently have its seat in the blood.

5. And now the surprising and epoch-making discovery was added that this resisting power, thus arti-

ficially developed in one animal, could, by the transfer of the blood, be transferred to another animal which was previously susceptible. Bacteriology having reached the stage of advancement that it had, it did not take long to settle the fact that this series of investigations had culminated in a most important practical discovery. It was fully demonstrated that a method, comparatively simple and apparently free from harm, had been found, by which animals could be protected against certain diseases, notably tetanus and diphtheria, and could with equal certainty be cured when those diseases had already entered the body.

The experiments upon human beings were then begun, at first upon a small scale, then more extensively, and with the results now known to all. This work has been done by scientists in a scientific spirit, and, to the credit of scientific medicine be it said, there is no secrecy and no degrading proprietorship in it.

Speaking now more particularly of diphtheria, the antitoxic serum is prepared as follows: Cultures of the most virulent diphtheria germs are allowed to grow in a fluid medium for several weeks. The fluid is now found to contain the diphtheria toxin, an intensely powerful poison. Small, non-fatal quantities of this toxin are injected into an animal, usually a horse. At intervals, of some days, progressively increasing quantities are injected, the result being the development of a correspondingly progressive resisting power in the animal. Finally, a condition is reached in which the animal is able to resist enormous quantities of the poison. The blood is now drawn, allowed to clot, the serum removed, and, after filtration and the addition of a small per cent. of antiseptic, is ready for use. This serum it is which seems to contain the antitoxic agent, and whose injection into a susceptible animal confers upon that animal, for a variable and limited time, the resisting power of the animal from which it was taken. This serum it is, also, which is injected into human beings exposed to or already sick with diphtheria.

I shall not now array the statistics which have been presented for and against this new treatment, which we owe chiefly to the labors of Behring and Kitasato in Germany, and Roux in France. Perhaps the most significant and most influential are those published by Virchow, summarizing the experience in the Emperor and Empress Frederic Hospital in Berlin. During a given period between five and six hundred cases of proven diphtheria were in the hospital. Of these over three hundred were treated with the serum, with a mortality of about 18 per cent. Over two hundred, treated without the serum, gave a mortality of about 47 per cent. Equally significant was the fact that when, at times, the serum treatment was suspended the mortality at once rose, to fall again promptly with the resumption of the antitoxin therapy. The known conservatism of Virchow

in such matters, together with his equally known
shrewdness as an observer, have therefore given much
weight to his favorable judgment of the treatment.
Theorizing, he says, must give way to the brute force
of these facts.

All of the experiments upon animals show that the
prophylactic powers of antitoxic serums is their greatest; that here their power is practically absolute; that
their curative power, also practically absolute in tetanus and diphtheria, is only absolute when applied
early in the course of the infection; that the quantity
of antitoxin necessary for prophylaxis or cure corre-
sponds to the quantity of toxin to be antagonized, and
finally, clinically considered, the longer the infection
has run and the more pronounced its character, the
larger is the dose of antitoxin necessary for cure.

Many questions have, of course, been raised as to
the limitations of the serum treatment and its possible
immediate or remote dangers. These questions will
require for their solution painstaking, accurate and
unprejudiced study, and we may be sure that the in-
exorable logic of time will give us the answer.

We have now passed through the period of acute,
intense interest. A world-wide experience with the
treatment has furnished the foundation for the necessary debate over the meaning and plan and value and
limitations of the therapeutic revolution which seems
upon us. We are now ready to settle down to a ju-
dicial frame of mind, to watch calmly the develop-

ment of events, and to do our part in the coming work. To this end two or three things are necessary:

First. Remembering that this new principle will doubtless be brought forward and is being brought forward in the treatment of other diseases, we must guard against hasty enthusiasms based upon insufficient scientific experiment, and we shall certainly have to guard against its commercial exploitation. Already, unless the signs are misleading, the latter evil is beginning to show itself. Plausible discoverers, with proprietary medicine schemes behind them, may create some stir among the unwary, for the nostrum business is at present flourishing even in the profession. But surely there ought not to be much difficulty in distinguishing science from mercenary trickery.

Second. We must expect and welcome and aid scientific investigation and experiment along these lines so clearly indicated as lines of progress.

Third. We must, while this whole matter is, as it is, in the experimental stage, keep a clear view of the facts, discriminating between things which are theoretical, uncertain and experimental, and those which are demonstrated beyond question. Speaking again of diphtheria only, the following seem to be the demonstrated facts which we must accept: That there is in this disease a germ which, being inoculated into animals, will kill them. That this germ, being artificially cultivated, gives rise to a toxic substance or

substances, which also will kill. That this germ or
this toxin, being introduced according to a certain
method and in progressive quantities into certain animals, there is developed in those animals a progressive resisting power to the germ or toxin, reaching an
astonishingly high degree, and lasting for a varying
but usually limited time. That the transfer of the
blood-serum of such animals to those previously susceptible to diphtheria does afford them almost at once
a practically absolute, though temporary, immunity
against or cure of diphtheria. That, in a word, it is
thus possible to absolutely control otherwise fatal experimental diphtheria intoxication and diphtheria infection in animals, and that without apparent harm.
That the longer the infection has run, the less certain
are the results, a point finally being reached when the
treatment may become impracticable and of little
avail. Experience with this treatment, applied to accidental human diphtheria, seems to indicate that human beings and the lower animals react in the same
way to the antitoxin serum therapy. But the truth
of this proposition is still to be fully and finally demonstrated. We must wait for the verdict of time before we can say of men as of animals: We know that
a specific for diphtheria has been found. While we
wait for and help to hasten the solution of the questions, let us hopefully keep in mind a clear view of
the established facts.

VIII

SERUM THERAPY IN DIPHTHERIA AND OTHER DISEASES.

THE passing year has been prolific of investigations and progress in the broadening field of bacteriology. More and more we see the study of the disease germs resulting in additions to our knowledge of diagnosis, treatment and prevention of the infectious processes. It is becoming more reliable and relied upon, in clinical as well as pathological diagnosis. It is becoming a more and more important part of sanitary science and preventive medicine. In the field of therapeutics it is opening up lines of investigation and experiment which are full of promise. No intelligent person any longer looks upon bacteriology as a fad or fashion. It has become in a hundred ways too well established and of too much practical value for any such view.

A year ago the subject of the antitoxin treatment and serum therapy was attracting universal attention and interest. Every one was watching it and eagerly asking what was to come of it. This interest, though quieter, is none the less intense, and current medical literature has fairly overflowed with discussions upon the new treatment as applied to several diseases, chiefly to diphtheria. It may be helpful to summarize briefly the best present views upon this subject. First, then, it appears to be generally agreed that diphtheria is a specific disease, due to a specific and recognizable microbe. The methods of recognizing and identifying this microbe have been well worked out, and it has therefore come to be relied upon as the most valuable because most positive means of diagnosis. The germ of diphtheria is one easily cultivated, and growing rapidly as it does, under proper conditions, its recognition may be made the basis of diagnosis for practical purposes. Diphtheria being a dangerous disease in a community, and its identification being of so much importance, health boards have in increasing numbers equipped themselves for doing this work in the interest and for the protection of the public health. Already at least two cities in Indiana have well-established departments in which the bacteriological diagnosis of diphtheria is made, and their results agree with those in other cities in testifying to its value and accuracy. No practicing physician who has once had within his reach and has made use of these aids to accuracy in his work will fail to appreciate the comforting assurance of their presence. No physician who has a few times experienced the relief of anxiety and uncertainty in doubtful cases will fail to acknowledge himself and his patients debtors to the science of bacteriology.

Second, the long-debated question of the relationship of diphtheria and membranous croup has been approaching a solution upon a basis which appears to be reliable. It does seem as though we should soon have a definite and positive answer to this vexed question. Extensive and accurate investigations have clearly proven that a large proportion—about 80 per cent.—of the cases ordinarily reported as membranous croup are membranous laryngitis, due to the poison of diphtheria. Acting, as they must, upon this demonstration, health boards are now coming to be almost unanimous in requiring a report of such cases, and in dealing with them as diphtheria. The presumption must be that at least the great majority of them are diphtheria. Clinical features, which still seem to sustain the doctrine of duality, there may be in some cases; but when from many of even such cases the microbes of diphtheria are obtained and being cultivated and inoculated, show their infectious quality, then, in the language of Virchow, as applied to antitoxin, theories must give way to the brute force of facts. Physicians, therefore, whatever their individual views as to membranous croup, should recognize the force of the facts, and should cheerfully support the health boards in following the course which is evidently the one of wisdom and safety.

At the same time it is to be said that, just as there are now known to be cases of membranous pharyngitis resembling diphtheria, but not due to the diph-

theria germ, so there may be, and probably are, cases
of membranous laryngitis non-diphtheritic in character.   And so the old question is not yet fully settled.
The immediate future, we can hardly doubt, will
bring the full and satisfactory solution.

As to the antitoxin treatment of diphtheria, the
writer feels disposed to give it a large place, since it
belongs now to both bacteriology and clinical medicine, though entirely an outgrowth of bacteriology.

In a former address emphasis was laid upon the importance of getting a clear view of the established
facts as distinguished from the theories, and of keeping these facts in mind as a guide to right-thinking
and acting.   At that time the things which we seemed
warranted in accepting as demonstrated were these:
that there is a germ in diphtheria, which, being inoculated in pure cultures, will kill; that this germ, being
artificially cultivated, produces an intense poison
which will kill; that, by the injection of gradually increasing quantities of this toxin into certain animals,
they may acquire an enormous resisting power to it
and to the germs; and that by the transfer of their
blood serum this resisting power might be transferred
for a limited time to other animals, and be for them
an almost specific preventative of diphtheria and almost equally specific cure of the disease in its earlier
stages.   These, which seemed worthy of acceptation
as demonstrated facts, remain as they were, though
their explanation still eludes us.

The chief theories in explanation of these facts are two: first, that there is in the antitoxin serum a substance which directly antagonizes the growth of the germs or neutralizes the toxin, or both; second, that its action is biological, rather than chemical, stimulating the body to an increased resistance. There are strong arguments in favor of each view, but we are not yet in a position to decide the question.

Meantime, the treatment has been applied in many thousands of cases, and what of the results? Statistics from many sources have been and are constantly being published, and of their value and significance others are as capable of judging as the writer. It must be said that the weight of opinion is in favor of the treatment. Certainly the majority of those who have used it extensively believe it to have given results surpassing those of anything heretofore known. Perhaps the best summary of the whole matter is that published by Welch, of Johns Hopkins University, and widely quoted. His conclusions are that the antitoxin is of great value, is comparatively harmless, and that it is our duty to use it. As a matter of record the following extract from Dr. Welch's paper is here given place:

In Dr. Welch's contribution, an analysis of 7,166 cases of antitoxin-treated diphtheria is reported from the hospitals of Germany, France, Austria and America. From a careful study of these cases, and from a thorough sifting of all the evidence, the figures show a mortality of 17.3 per cent.

Alongside of these cases, and in the same hospitals, with the same favorable surroundings, 5,706 cases of diphtheria were treated by the old method, with a death-rate of 42.1 per cent.

"There was, therefore," says Dr. Welch, "an apparent reduction of case mortality by the use of antitoxin of 55.8 per cent."

Statistics, according to the age of the patient, both with and without the serum treatment, afford very interesting reading.

From a summary of this table, Welch says: "Of 1,729 cases of diphtheria with a fatality of 14.9 per cent., 1,115 cases treated with antitoxin during the first three days of the disease yielded a fatality of 8.5 per cent., whereas 546 cases in which antitoxin was first injected after the third day of the disease yielded a fatality of 27.8 per cent.

"Of 232 in which treatment was begun on the first day five died, or 2.15 per cent. Of 492 cases in which treatment was begun on the second day 30 died, 7.7 per cent. Of 331 cases in which treatment was begun on the third day 43 died, 13 per cent.; on the fourth day 19 per cent., on the fifth day 39.3 per cent., on the sixth day 34.1 per cent."

In closing his report Dr. Welch makes this statement: "The principal conclusion which I would draw from this paper is that our study of the results of the treatment of over 7,000 cases of diphtheria by the antitoxin demonstrates beyond all doubt that antidiphtheritic serum is a specific curative agent for diphtheria, surpassing in its efficacy all other known methods of treatment for this disease."

There are occasional unpleasant effects in the form of more or less intense erythema, sometimes with fever, severe pains, glandular swellings, and even effusions into joints or serous cavities. A few serious accidents and even deaths have followed the antitoxin, and apparently due to the injections. Just what these accidents mean, and whether they are inseparable from the antitoxic serum, we do not know, but they serve to make us properly cautious, and warn us not to accept too readily the assurance that, even under the most extreme precautions of preparation, such an agent is always and wholly free from danger. The good appears to overbalance any evil, but we are not yet sure that there is no possibility of harm.

Diphtheria is not the only disease in which antitoxic serum therapy has been applied. The principles of production and use being established, the endeavor is constantly being made to extend its sphere. Indeed, the tetanus antitoxin preceded that of diphtheria, and in animals experimented upon in the laboratory seems to have been equally successful. For obvious reasons, however, its clinical application has not been as extensive nor apparently of as much value. A tetanus antitoxin is now within the reach of physicians and is certainly worthy of trial, at least in the early stages of lockjaw. According to all who have had experience with it, it must be given in large doses and as early as possible in the disease. If possible, it should be used as a preventive after a suspicious injury.

For pneumonia, typhoid fever and tuberculosis, antitoxic serums have been prepared and have been used in a considerable number of cases, and in several other diseases they have been and are being tried to a limited extent. It is too early to form any reliable opinion as to the value of the treatment in these diseases. The serum treatment of tuberculosis has been given a sufficient trial to indicate that, as at present prepared, not much can be expected from it.

As to tuberculosis, the greatest of the serious diseases with which we have to deal, each passing year is bringing out in bolder lines the proof of its infectious character. Personally, the writer grows more and more convinced of the truth of this view, and of the importance of action based thereupon. Of this he has something to say elsewhere.

Cholera has been the subject of a large amount of investigation, the result of which has been to emphasize its water-born character in many if not most instances, and to make easier and more reliable the bacteriological diagnosis. The preventive inoculations against cholera have been carried out upon a larger scale by Haffkine in India. His recent report is a model of scientific spirit and work, and appears to justify a hopeful view of the measure. His investigations will be continued under government aid, and we shall look with interest for the publication of results from time to time.

The injection of the erysipelas toxin in malignant disease has been continued by many observers in this country and in Europe. It still appears from this experience that the treatment does have considerable retarding or curative effect in sarcoma, but little if any in carcinoma. In general, however, there seems to be less promise in the measure than a year ago.

The influenza bacillus seems to have established itself in the opinion of most bacteriologists as the true germ of la grippe, and several observers have expressed a high opinion of its diagnostic value.

The subject of cancer and its possible microbic origin has engaged the attention of many investigators, and various claims to a discovery of the specific causative agent have been made. But most of the so-called cancer germs have been shown to be only bodies appearing during and resulting from the normal or abnormal cellular changes which occur in or about the growth. The germ of cancer, if such exist, has not yet found an established place in bacteriology. From the far west, from the rising empire of Japan, comes the news confirming that announced before, that Kitasato had discovered, cultivated and proven the specific character of the microbe of the bubonic plague, which has raged in China during the last two years.   And thus another mark of honor has been won by the already famous Japanese, who a few years ago was a favorite pupil and assistant of Koch in Berlin.   And thus, too, peace and science have their victories there as well as war.

IX.

THE POSITION OF VACCINATION IN PATHOLOGY AND BACTERIOLOGY.

IT is not the chief purpose of this paper to enter into a direct argument upon the protective influence of vaccination against smallpox, nor to array the statistics in its favor. Such an effort would surely be superfluous. He who in this day, with the light of the last decade's revelations before him, issues broad denials of the efficacy of vaccination, seriously compromises his reputation for professional and scientific sanity. It were useless to argue with him. But in view of the recent advances in our knowledge of the infectious diseases, and the efforts being made to extend the range of preventive and curative inoculations, it may be of interest and profit to survey the field and see just where vaccination against smallpox stands in pathology, what it means, its extent and limitations, and what its promise for success in other diseases.

Two theories have always existed, and do, to some extent, still exist, as to the nature of cowpox. The one, that it is a peculiar, distinct disease, whose antag-

99

onism to smallpox is likewise a peculiar, isolated fact,
an exotic in the field of pathology. The other, that
it is simply smallpox in the cow, and vaccination simply the induction of a modified form of smallpox.
Either of these theories might be true and yet the protective influence of vaccination not excite, in this day,
great incredulity among scientific men. For, sup-
posing the former theory correct, it has been shown
that there is an antagonism between certain distinct
bacteria, an antagonism so pronounced as to be inhib-
itory or destructive. Thus the intensely malignant
anthrax is prevented or arrested by simultaneous inoculation with the comparatively harmless bacillus prodigiosus. There are other antagonisms of a similar
character, though perhaps none equally striking. It
is, therefore, quite within reason, and within the
sphere of analogy, to suppose that cowpox, being a distinct disease, might protect from smallpox.

But credible though it may be, and quite within
the range of possibility, there seems really little now
left in support of this theory of cowpox. The facts
of nature, i. e., the natural history of cowpox, the increased knowledge of recent years in the whole field
of bacterial pathology, and direct experiment, combine to strengthen the view that cowpox is simply
bovine smallpox.

If this is true, the whole matter becomes a simple
one.

Discovered accidentally, but worked out by the

painstaking and lifetime devotion of Jenner, and to his immortal renown, vaccination was for a long time thought to occupy a peculiar and isolated place in pathology. The mystery about it, and that which strengthened incredulity as to the identity of cowpox and smallpox, was this:—how can such a virulent disease as smallpox be so modified and mollified by passing through the body of the cow? For such a thing there was no analogy.

But the investigations of the last ten years have put an entirely new face upon this idol of unbelief. The modification of a disease by passing it through the body of certain animals has become a commonplace matter in pathology. We no longer wonder at such a claim nor doubt its possibility.

It is unnecessary to enter into the details of these new facts, they are so generally known. It is sufficient to refer to the modification of the virus of rabies, of the pneumococcus and of others, brought about by this means, or by other methods of altering the culture soil or the conditions of growth.

Acting upon the view that cowpox was modified smallpox, the attempt has been repeatedly made to imitate the whole process artificially; that is, to secure vaccine virus by inoculating the cow with smallpox. The first to do this is supposed to have been Gassner of Gunzburg (1807). It was done on a large scale by Thiele of Kasan and Ceely of England (1838). They carried their vaccine virus, thus obtained, through sixty to seventy generations in several thousand persons, and subsequently proved its efficiency by repeated inoculations with genuine variola humana. (Whittaker.) Similar experiments were made by Badcock and Seufft. The committees of Lyons (1865) and Turin (1874) opposed these conclusions, but they failed to explain the facts. The whole subject has recently been gone over by an English experimenter, who shows how those committees were misled, and claims to have finally settled the matter.

We have doubtless something still to learn about the methods of securing vaccine matter by the inoculation of animals with human variola. Perhaps the best results will only be got by using other animals as well as the cow; perhaps we shall have to wait for the discovery of the smallpox germ and the more exact experiments which would follow. In the meantime we must admit the strength of the evidence that cowpox is a modification of smallpox, and that vaccination is simply variolation in mild and modified form; that it is inoculation stripped of its virulence and dangers.

Vaccination, in the light of modern knowledge, takes its proper place, falling naturally and easily under the sway of those principles which rule in the field of pathology in which it belongs.

What are some of these principles revealed by a study of that great group of diseases, one attack of which affords immunity?

First. The immunity or protection afforded by one attack of a disease is not necessarily absolute.

Illustrations of this rule are met with in our daily practice. Thus, we see those who have unquestionably had cholera, typhoid fever or scarlatina, suffering from second or even third attacks. This is true also of smallpox. Such experiences are exceptions, rare exceptions with some diseases, but they occur with sufficient frequency to warn us against too radical views of the value of acquired immunity, while they in no way disprove the fact of such immunity.

Second. The protection afforded by one attack of a disease is not necessarily permanent.

That the protective influence of the primary attack fades with the lapse of time is, with some diseases, a matter of common observation. The duration of the immunity varies within wide limits. With some maladies it is practically life-long; with others so short as to be, to ordinary experience, hardly discernible. The difficulty of defining these limits is increased by the necessity of including in the calculation that peculiar insusceptibility to certain diseases which seems to be gradually and naturally acquired with advancing years. In this connection we must, however, not forget the havoc wrought, even among the adult population, with the advent of a new disease. The Sandwich Islands were swept, as by a hurricane, by the fatal breath of measles in 1848, while the Fiji Islanders fled in terror from its deadly presence.

Modern bacteriological experiment has stepped in at this point to enlarge our knowledge, revealing the fact that some diseases are followed by a period of immunity, distinct, but so short-lived as to have escaped observation or demonstration. This seems to be true of cholera. From such short periods we rise, step by step, to reach diseases like measles, scarlatina, typhoid and variola, the protection of which usually extends over such a time as spans the ordinary duration of human life. Fortunate it is that immunity is so often long-continued. Yet the fact remains that, as a general rule, with passing years its energy declines.

When we come to apply this rule to vaccination, we shall see how the recognition but misunderstanding of it at one time threatened to wreck that life-saving agency.

Third. Quantity and quality of the virus, or vigor of the attack, is an important factor in the immunity which shall follow.

It is a common opinion, both professional and popular, that those who have experienced mild attacks of a disease are more liable to recurrence than those in whom the attack has been pronounced. Laboratory experiment has again stepped in here with a contribution of more exact knowledge. It has been abundantly shown in the laboratory, where the conditions can be so thoroughly controlled, that the quantity and activity of the virus or other protective agent stand usually in direct ratio to the immunity which such treatment affords. Thus Pasteur's first vaccine affords but feeble protection, the second vaccine increases the security; and so advancing, step by step, from weaker to stronger virus, practically absolute protection against rabies is secured to animals.

Fourth. The protection afforded by one attack of a disease is a positive, an active thing; it is an endowment with a new power.

He who has not had measles, scarlatina nor variola is susceptible to those diseases. In no other known way can he obtain an immunity. If this statement seems trite and unworthy of the prominence here given it, the justification will be found in its important bearing upon the practical application of vaccination.

If now these principles are correct, they ought to be applicable to vaccination.

First, we should not expect the protection thus afforded to be absolute. Experience alone could decide the matter. And experience leaves us with a trifle of uncertainty, because the immunity approaches so near to completeness that we can but suspect that the few exceptions are only apparent and due to some defect in the vaccination. Those few persons who have had variola within a few years of vaccination may and probably have not had a genuine inoculation with cowpox. But, it need hardly be said, the departure from complete protection is so slight as to be of small practical moment.

Second, we should not expect the protection of vaccination to be permanent; certainly not in view of the fact that unmodified smallpox itself does not always afford permanent safety. Jenner himself erred at this point, believing that cowpoxing protected for life, and we can easily understand how he made this mistake. With the light of modern knowledge, still more with the light of a century's experience before us, we can easily pardon an error into which he fell simply from lack of experience which could only come with the lapse of years. He did not live long enough to get a final view of the matter. When, with passing years, some of those who had been vaccinated began to show a susceptibility to smallpox, and the truth which is so clear to us began to force itself upon the world, it came with such a shock as almost to threaten, as I have said, the ruin of vaccination. The suspicion arose and was industriously fostered that the whole thing was a gigantic and astounding delusion. Fortunately, calmer minds saw the true state of the matter, with the result that the necessity for and the practice of re-vaccination became established.

While it is evidently impossible to fix upon a time at which the efficacy of vaccination has declined to the danger point, there is a substantial agreement among all authorities which, being acted upon, leads to almost assured safety. The German statistics thoroughly and accurately collected seem to show that no case of smallpox has occurred in that country within ten years of a successful vaccination. This is coming to be accepted throughout the world as the basis for the regulation of re-vaccination. If all children were vaccinated within the first and at the tenth year of life, smallpox would be practically abolished, as indeed it has been from those communities in which this rule is followed.

Third, we should expect the thoroughness of the vaccination to stand in something like a direct ratio to the degree of protection. And this we certainly find to be true. The experience in every outbreak of smallpox confirms this rule. And the lesson of it is obvious: we should vaccinate thoroughly, knowing that the result will be a proportionate thoroughness of protection. We wrong those who commit this matter to our care, and wrong the public, by failure to appreciate and act upon this too much neglected truth.

Fourth, the protection afforded by vaccination is a positive, an active thing; it is an endowment with a new power, conferred upon the individual and to be obtained, so far as we know, only in this way. He who has not had variola is susceptible to that disease unless properly vaccinated. And that vaccination should be genuine.

The protection comes, not by the scarification and its resulting lesion, not by the scarification and the application of vaccine lymph; but by the successful induction of the specific lesions of vaccinia, and the vaccinator should see to it that this is secured or the procedure repeated. Many of those said to have been vaccinated have doubtless not been really vaccinated at all. Thus, in the presence of smallpox, discredit is thrown upon vaccination and danger upon the community.

The public should be made to understand this: that the vaccinator should have full opportunity to insure genuine vaccinations, and that the security arising out of the new comparative rarity of smallpox may be a false security unless reinforced by genuine, general, and repeated endowment with that active power of resistance which can come only in one way.

In a word, the public should distinctly understand that the immunity through vaccination, though practically complete, is temporary and must be reinforced by repetition; that the process must be genuine, and that, somewhat unpleasant though it may be, it should be thorough. With these injunctions may happily be joined the assurance of safety by their observance.

In conclusion, something ought to be said, from a pathological standpoint, about the supposed dangers of vaccination. Whatever ground there may have been for fear in its earlier history, when the human lymph was indiscriminately used, vaccination as at present practiced is attended by but trifling danger. Outcries to the contrary, with the wild statements which sometimes accompany them, are but the wanderings of distorted vision and disordered minds.

The dangers of vaccination, such as there are, arise from four sources:

1. The induction of a very mild infectious disease.

2. The transfer of human disease by the use of human lymph. Of these syphilis is the most to be feared. There are others, but of much less importance. This is avoided by the use of animal virus.

3. The possible transfer of diseases to which the animal is subject. Among these, theory, or more frequently perhaps imagination, suggests many; facts point to but few, such as erysipelas and suppuration. This danger is reduced to almost nothing by proper care in the management of the vaccine stables.

4. The vaccination wound may become infected, as may any other trifling abrasion. Suppuration or erysipelas may supervene and cause trouble, but the avoidance of these complications is so plain and simple, in this day of surgical cleanliness, as to hardly need mention.

There remains, perhaps, after all, a minute but real danger, which, though not for a moment to be placed in the balance over against the incalculable good, cannot be finally ruled out till the discovery of the specific bacteria of vaccination enables us to handle and apply the virus with the exactness of a chemical experiment. In the meantime we may rest assured, and may assure the public in whose interests alone we are working, that the dangers of vaccination are to-day almost entirely imaginary and hardly worth more than a passing thought, and are chiefly of historical interest. For the distorted and extreme statements which are sometimes issued, there is, in the face of the plain facts of experience and of science, no excuse. It is hardly too much to say that they are a criminal abuse of privilege.

In this day the public has not the fear of smallpox before its eyes as formerly. It forgets too easily. We have no realizing sense of its horrors. Therefore we see growing a false sense of security and a growing carelessness in regard to the necessity and the means of insuring safety. If we will only follow the plain teachings of that which has now become an integral part of biological science, availing ourselves of the equally plain lessons of experience in its application, we need have no fears of the "stinking pestilence" which struck terror to the hearts of our forefathers. The truth is before us, and the truth will make us safe. If we grow too careless, indifferent and neglectful, history may repeat itself in giving another and a different lesson from experience.

From such a lesson we may well pray, in the name of Jenner, to be delivered.

X.

BACTERIA, AND BACTERIOLOGICAL METHODS AND DIAGNOSIS.

BACTERIA are minute cells, classified biologically far down the line in the vegetable kingdom. They vary much in size, but all are so small as to be beyond the range of unaided vision. An ordinary-sized bacterium would be one ten-thousandth to one twenty-thousandth of an inch in diameter or length. When seen singly, they are practically colorless, but many bacteria, when growing in masses or colonies, present distinct and even brilliant colors. Such colonies often resemble, in gross appearance, the ordinary moulds.

While bacteria are so numerous and widespread as to be commonly said to be ubiquitous, it is not true, as many believe, that the air is swarming with them. Like all bodies of greater specific gravity than air, they tend to settle, so that the quiet atmosphere in many places is comparatively free from microbes. Exposed waters, the surface and the upper layers of the soil, and the surfaces of solid bodies generally, harbor bacteria in large numbers; but the deeper layers of the soil, the waters from clean springs, and deep wells free from surface drainage, are comparatively or quite sterile. The unexposed tissues of healthy bodies are also normally free from germs.

Though it is now known that many diseases are caused by bacteria, it must not be supposed that all the bacteria are enemies of the higher forms of life. On the contrary, many of them play a beneficent role in promoting the disintegration of dead organic material, which would otherwise, by accumulation, make the world one vast graveyard; in preparing, by such changes, the food for other living beings, and in rendering the soil suitable for the growth of higher plants. We fear the microbes which produce disease, yet life would soon be impossible to higher organisms without the helpful work of others. In all our study of bacteria let us not forget that they may be the friends as well as the enemies of mankind. It is, however, the disease-producing micro-organisms which engage the chief study of the physician, for these it is with which he has to contend. These it is of whose presence he must learn, in the field of diagnosis, to be forewarned.

The bacteria, like other living things, perform the ordinary functions of life. They breathe; they eat, taking in food substances, changing, digesting and appropriating them to their needs, excreting the waste products. They multiply and reproduce their kind. Like other living beings, also, their existence, and especially their growth and multiplication, is chiefly under the control of four factors, namely, food, temperature, moisture, and the presence or absence of air. And again like most other living beings, the evidence of their activity is not chiefly mechanical, but is found in the field of biological chemistry.

Many bacteria grow at the ordinary temperature of the house or the surrounding air, while some require for their multiplication temperatures approximating that of the bodies of warm-blooded animals. They do not multiply in the dried state, being in this respect again like other seeds. Some require while some reject a free access of air. Some welcome while some quickly die under direct sunlight. Indeed, the more we study them the more clearly do we see that they are under the laws which prevail throughout the organic world.

The attempt to classify the bacteria on a strictly scientific, that is, a botanical basis, has thus far been unsatisfactory. They are therefore classified according to certain of their more conspicuous characteristics. Of these groupings the most common, and the one generally used, is that based upon their form. According to this system we describe most bacteria as belonging to one or the other of three great groups. These are: the round organisms or micrococci, the rod-shaped organisms or bacilli, and those having a spiral or corkscrew shape, called spirilla. Thus we speak of the micrococci of erysipelas, the bacilli of diphtheria, and the spirilla of cholera. The term bacterium, though originally given to the rod or staff-like forms, has now come to be applied to micro-organisms or germs in general.

Another important classification of bacteria is based upon some marked biological property or activity. Thus are described the color-producing or chromogenic organisms; the saprophytes, or those which live upon dead organic material; the saprogenic or putrefaction-producing bacteria; the zymogenic or ferment producers, and hence the old term zymotic or ferment diseases; and finally, to the physician the most important of all, the pathogenic or disease-producing microbes. Flourescent and phosphorescent bacteria are also described. These terms and groups are not mutually exclusive, since, for example, bacteria may be pathogenic and at the same time chromogenic or color-producing. According to their ability to grow with or without free oxygen, micro-organisms are also said to be aerobic or anaerobic, a classification of great practical as well as scientific importance.

Many, perhaps most, bacteria are motionless, save for a fine vibratory activity, the molecular or so-called Brownian movement. Others have the power of true locomotion, due to vigorous contractions and expansions of their bodies, or to the possession of minute appendages called flagella. At best, however, the sphere of such locomotion is limited, and does not confer the power of passing over great distances. Any considerable migration of bacteria within the body is brought about only by transport through the various body fluids.

Bacteria multiply by the process of fission or splitting, one cell, by this simple process, giving rise to two, four or more daughter cells, which have or soon assume all of the properties of the parent. In addition to this process of splitting, they reproduce themselves by spore or seed formation, one cell giving rise to one spore, the latter proceeding at once to develop into a mature bacterium, or lying dormant until the conditions for its full development are present. As a rule, these spores are much more tenacious of life than the mature bacteria, are much more resistant to hostile influences, and therefore more independent of their environment. For these reasons spores will often resist drying, and degrees of cold and heat, even to freezing, or boiling for a time, such as would rapidly destroy the fully developed organisms. In this spore stage, bacteria, like other seeds, may frequently retain their life, while not growing nor multiplying, for long periods. Such facts often explain the insidious persistence of infectious material even under apparently adverse conditions. The seeds of various grains lie dry and cold in the bin during the winter, ready to sprout with the advent of spring. And so with the seeds of disease.

Various theories have been proposed to explain the disease-producing activity of micro-organisms. Most

of these theories have some measure of truth, but all
have failed, until recently, to explain the facts. The
problem has now been worked out to a fairly satisfactory conclusion in the establishment of the toxin
theory. We now know that most of the results of
bacterial action are explained by the production in
the course of their growth of certain new substances.
If these substances are injurious or poisonous to the
living body, the bacteria producing them are said to
be toxic; if they are produced during the growth of
the microbes within the living body, such microbes
are said to be infectious. If the toxin-forming organisms are regularly associated as causative agents with
a peculiar or specific disease, they are called specific
bacteria. Thus the definition and classification of
many diseases has become more accurate, more rational, because built more nearly upon the basis of
causation. Infectious diseases are those which are
caused by the presence and growth, within the body,
of living producers of poisons. Specific infectious
diseases are those each of which is caused by a particular living toxin-producer, a particular or specific
bacterium. For example, the condition commonly
known as blood-poisoning may be due to any of a
number of bacteria, while the peculiar and specific disease diphtheria, with its peculiar poisoning of the
blood, is believed to be caused by the specific diphtheria bacillus alone. An important corollary to such
a doctrine is found in this: that if, for example, the

latter statement is true, we have in the detection of
the diphtheria bacillus a positive means of recognizing or diagnosing diphtheria, and we at once begin to
see how the science of bacteriology becomes a part of
everyday practical medicine.

Bacteriology has entered into and become a working part of practical medicine in several ways. It
suggests and directs general preventive measures
against the infectious diseases. It suggests and
guides preventive and curative measures in individual
cases; and it is affording us more accurate and more
rapid means of diagnosis in an increasing number of
diseases. It is therefore becoming of importance to
every practicing physician, and of interest to every intelligent person, to know something of the methods of
bacteriological work, especially of that part of it
which is applicable in the working laboratory—that
is, in the consulting room of the doctor. The more
this work is studied the more will it appear that it
follows in many respects the principles and methods
of ordinary agriculture. Keeping this fact in mind,
many otherwise strange things become clear and
simple.

The cultivation of bacteria has, mainly through the
efforts of a few great men like Pasteur and Koch, become a comparatively simple matter, now taught in
every well-equipped medical school. In the earlier
days it was customary to cultivate bacteria in fluids,
such as beef broth. But with this method it is diffi-

cult to separate the different varieties which grow in
confusion in the liquid. The invention by Koch of
the solid culture soil has made the separation of micro-
organisms rapid and, as a rule, easy. The substances
used for this purpose have been many, but experience
has singled out a few which answer all ordinary purposes. The simplest of these is the surface of a
cooked potato, upon which many bacteria may be sat-
isfactorily grown. But the potato has been largely
superseded by culture soils or media having an albuminous basis, such as that derived from meat. In
order to solidify this meat extract or bouillon, about
10 per cent. of gelatin is added, giving a clear, firm
product, the beef-gelatin soil. But since gelatin soft-
ens at the body or incubator temperature, it has in
recent years been improved upon by the use of an
Asiatic sea-weed called agar-agar. This substance, of
which about 2 per cent. is added to the bouillon, gives
us the now widely used beef-agar culture medium,
having the great advantage of remaining solid at the
heat of the body and of the incubator. It therefore
serves for the cultivation of bacteria which require
such temperatures for their successful growth. In
order to retain as much as possible of the albuminous
constituents of the beef after the repeated heating
necessary in its preparation, it is either peptonized or
artificially digested, or pre-digested albumen in the
form of peptone is added. If to this peptonized beef-
agar 4 or 5 per cent. of glycerin be added, its field of

usefulness is widened, since upon this medium will
grow well certain bacteria which grow but indiffer-
ently or not at all upon the simpler soils.

In his researches upon the tubercle bacillus Koch
brought forward solidified blood-serum, which has
proven the most valuable culture medium for some of
the sensitive or the strongly parasitic microbes. It
was upon this substance that he was first able to grow
the germ of tuberculosis, and, as a result, to work out
the perplexing problem of the cause of this disease.

Certain fluids obtained from the living body are
sometimes used alone or in combination as culture
media. Such are the liquid exudates in cases of
pleurisy, peritonitis, or other inflammations of serous
membranes. Finally, the living body is itself made
to do service as a laboratory for the growth of bacteria, thus imitating exactly the natural process.

Of all of these substances, those most frequently
used are the glycerin-agar, and the solidified blood-
serum, either pure or variously modified. The blood-
serum and agar are often combined with happy results.

In all culture work absolute sterilization of materials and instruments is necessary, lest slight contamination at the beginning grow into gross and misleading contamination at the end. If we are to in-
terpret correctly the final findings, we must know with
certainty the beginning. There must be in our final
cultures no bacteria except those placed there at the
start.

The sterilization of culture materials and apparatus is accomplished by heat, either dry or moist, according to the character of the substance to be sterilized. For this purpose two pieces of apparatus have come into use: the steam sterilizer, similar to an ordinary steam cooker, and the dry sterilizer, a simple portable sheet-iron oven. The culture medium is placed in sterilized vessels, usually ordinary chemists' glass test tubes, the mouths of which are tightly filled with cotton, the latter having been previously subjected to heat in the oven. Access of air is thus allowed, while bacteria are effectually excluded. Open vessels, which cannot be plugged with cotton, are placed under a belljar inverted over a plate of glass, the whole constituting what is called a moist chamber, in which the growing cultures may be inspected. Other vessels of special construction are used for special purposes, but the test-tube method of culture is the one followed in all ordinary work. If the tubes are to be kept for some time either in the open air or in the incubator, drying of their contents is prevented by rubber caps placed over the cotton plug. The whole process is indeed similar to that of cooking, sealing, and thus preserving fruit. For the cultivation of bacteria at the body temperature an incubating or breeding oven is used, similar to, though more accurately constructed than, the ordinary egg hatcher. This apparatus is a double-walled, felt-jacketed oven, the space between the walls being filled with water to insure against rapid fluctuations of temperature. It is heated by a self-regulating gas burner, so that the temperature is maintained for days or weeks at the desired point. Many bacteria which grow best and most rapidly in the incubator may also be successfully though more slowly and somewhat imperfectly grown without any special incubating apparatus, provided the temperature be kept fairly near that of the body.

Inoculation of bacteria-containing material onto the culture medium is usually made with a platinum or other wire, sterilized before and immediately after use by heating in a clean flame. In rapidity of growth bacteria vary, like other seeds, and under similar conditions. If the conditions are favorable, most bacteria present visible cultures in from one to three or four days. A few of the known varieties require from one to three weeks for their development.

To illustrate the method of bacteriological investigation in its simplest form, let us suppose that we wish to discover the germ of diphtheria. Having prepared the culture material and been assured, by protracted observation, of its freedom from bacterial growth, we take upon a sterilized wire from the throat a little of the membrane presumed to contain the specific germ. Removing for a moment the cotton plug from a tube, this material is deposited in the previously warmed and liquefied agar-glycerin. The contents of this tube, or of another into which a portion has been transferred from the first for the purpose of dilution,

is now poured upon a sterilized plate of glass, where it
quickly hardens into a transparent film resembling
gelatin. Placing this plate in the moist chamber,
and enclosing the whole in the incubator, we await
the resulting culture. After some days we find the
plate studded with bacterial colonies of various appearance. Ocular and microscopic examination of
these colonies reveals the fact that several varieties of
microbes were present in the throat and are growing
on the plate. Repeating the procedure, we make
plate cultures from the different colonies, each succeeding experiment affording more nearly a pure culture of one variety. Finally, we reach, upon different plates, pure cultures of each variety of micro-organism which grew upon the first plate. One of
these we presume to be the germ of diphtheria. We
now proceed to test the presumption. Animals are
inoculated with each variety of bacterium, the one
which produces diphtheria in the animal being now,
with stronger conviction, believed to be the one sought
for. Carefully studying this germ and recording the
results of the study, we go back and repeat a number
of times the whole procedure. We examine many
cases of diphtheria and identify this germ in all. We
thus prove its constant presence in the disease. We
re-cultivate it and repeat many times the successful
inoculations, finding it always present in the artifi-
cially-produced disease; and thus we complete the
chain of proof and the identification of the germ of

diphtheria. Having done this, we are able to identify it at any time or place, and, by recognizing it, to diagnose the disease to which it belongs.

Were the attempt to identify the germ of each specific infectious disease so easily carried to a successful issue, little would now remain to be done in this direction. Unfortunately, the task is not usually so simple. Difficulties or temporary defeats are likely to be met with at every step. To begin with, the material taken from the throat, though containing various bacteria, might not include the germ of diphtheria. The final inoculation experiments would therefore be negative. Or the culture soil might not be suitable for this particular microbe, and again the results would be negative. Unfavorable conditions, such as the presence or absence of air, might defeat the experiment; or the growth of one or more of the other bacteria might obscure, retard or prevent the growth of those sought for. Finally, though the desired germ might be obtained in pure culture, the animals experimented upon might not be susceptible to the disease in question, and again a negative or neutral result would be reached. Here, therefore, as in agriculture, though the general principles and methods be simple, a reliable conclusion is to be reached only by a successful management of details. But having once identified a germ and demonstrated its specific causative relation to a disease, its identification and manipulation thereafter usually becomes comparatively easy, and the way opens for experiments with it in the direction of diagnosis, prevention and cure.

It has already been pointed out that the explanation of the disease-producing action of bacteria is to be sought chiefly in their poisonous contents and products. For the purpose of obtaining these poisonous products or toxins for experimental work, the bacteria, once obtained in pure cultures, are usually grown in liquids. The bacteria are then filtered out by porcelain filters, leaving a fluid containing the toxin, which, representing the active principles of the bacteria, may, for experimental purposes, be used in exact dosage. Or, to more fully imitate nature, the bacteria themselves, washed free from all extraneous substances, may be pulverized and dissolved to obtain their constituents. Here again, while general principles and methods are simple, the details of successful work are often many and perplexing. But such difficult procedures belong chiefly in the experimental laboratory; the culture work available and useful to the practicing physician, following, as it does, the paths laid out by the investigators, once learned, is uncomplicated and easy.

The microscopic study of bacteria is an exceedingly attractive subject to the physician, revealing a world of curious and interesting things, and opening up a most valuable field of diagnosis. Improvements in the construction and manipulation of the microscope have brought the bacteria within the reach of our vision. A brief description of this part of bacteriological work will therefore not be amiss, especially since it has become of everyday utility.

In preparing for the microscopic examination of bacteria the following steps are taken with all fluid or semi-fluid specimens. A minute portion of an artificial culture or of the microbe-containing material is spread in a very thin layer upon a slide or cover glass. This is allowed to dry in the air, or is dried by gentle heating. When dry, it is passed, prepared-side upward, three or four times through the clean flame of a spirit lamp or Bunsen burner. This coagulates uniformly the albumen and cements the specimen to the glass, and it is now ready for the important process of staining. If the bacteria are to be inspected in their natural condition, unstained, they are placed in a drop of distilled water and immediately examined. Thus seen, the germs are almost or quite colorless. It is therefore customary to give to them an artificial coloring in order to render them more visible and their outlines, and to some extent their structure, more distinct. For this purpose solutions of the basic anilin dyes are generally used. Among these are two which have been settled upon as answering all ordinary demands. These are a red and a blue dye, named respectively fuchsin and methyl blue. Solutions of these colors are made in water or alcohol, or in both, and to these

solutions are sometimes added certain substances
which increase their power of staining. Most of the
known bacteria may be stained by exposure for a few
seconds or minutes to a simple watery solution of one
of these anilin dyes. The process may be hastened
or intensified or made applicable to otherwise resist-
ent organisms by heating the solution. If the bacteria still resist the dye, it may be made to "bite" into
them by the addition of mordants, such as anilin oil,
carbolic acid, or caustic potash, following the methods
used in the dyeing of cloth. The most vigorous
staining effects are secured by hot solutions containing such mordants, and thus only are certain bacteria
successfully colored. Spores are, as a rule, more resistant to staining than the mature bacteria. A special method of staining is that of Gram, in which
iodine dissolved in potassium iodide solution is used to
protect from decolorization certain bacteria which
have once been stained. The reaction of bacteria to
this method of staining having been determined, it
subsequently serves as an aid in identifying them.
Decolorizing agents, water, alcohol, and mineral acids,
are used when desirable, to remove an excess or all of
the dye from stained bacteria. All stained specimens
are washed in water before examining them. The
behavior of microbes under the influence of the
stronger decolorizing solutions is sometimes of much
significance in distinguishing them from others similar in appearance. This is an essential feature of the

process by which the tubercle bacilli are recognized
for diagnostic purposes. Spores usually require the
application of the more energetic staining processes,
and resist the action of decolorizing agents more than
mature bacteria. The staining of bacteria in thin
sections of tissue is accomplished by the method just
described, but requires more time, more care in the
use of decolorizing agents, and often contrast colors
for the tissue. For the latter purpose we use one of
the acid anilin dyes, such as eosin, or a tissue stain like
carmine or hematoxylin. Double staining is the
process of giving one color to one variety of bacteria
and another contrast color to the others or to the surrounding field. It is often of aid to the eye in locat-
ing and distinguishing a particular variety under the
microscope.

To illustrate these processes we prepare a number
of specimens upon thin cover glasses, spreading, drying and heating them so that all are ready for staining. We now test upon them the dyes prepared as
described above, a few drops of staining solution being placed upon each glass. After a few minutes the
glasses are washed in water, the clean faces are wiped
dry, and they are ready for inspection. The first
specimens have been subjected to a cold watery solution of the dye. Examination shows most of the bacteria to have taken up the color. Several varieties remain colorless. A repetition of the process, except
that the glasses are held in forceps, prepared-side up-

ward, over a flame till the solution steams, reveals but
few varieties unstained. Again we stain a similar
series, using a cold solution containing 5 per cent. of
carbolic acid, repeating the procedure with the same
solution heated, and with solutions, cold and hot, containing a minute quantity of potassium hydrate. In
the last specimens, stained with the mordants, we shall
probably find all the different varietis to have taken
up the dye.

If now we subject all of these specimens for a few
seconds to a 25 per cent. solution of nitric acid, the
color, as seen by the unaided eye, fades from all.
Microscopic examination shows that almost all of the
bacteria have been decolorized by the acid. One or
two varieties only retain the stain, standing out con-
spicuously colored upon a colorless background.
Upon close study these will probably be found to be
just the ones which resisted the simpler staining, requiring the most energetic dyes. The tubercle bacillus, for instance, stains with difficulty, but, once colored, it resists the decolorizing agent to which most
others succumb. Selecting such a specimen, we stain
it again, after thorough washing to remove the acid,
with a watery solution of a contrast color. The resistant bacteria do not take the dye, while other bacteria, mucus, and debris, making up the field, do.
The former present the one color, the latter the other.
And thus we see illustrated the selective action of the
dyes, and the staining and decolorizing reaction of

bacteria. In a score of ways these reactions may be used in the staining and identification of disease germs. It is fortunate that this is true, for thus only is made easy and of everyday value the identification of certain microbes the recognition of which would otherwise require the more difficult and tedious processes of culture and inoculation.

For the examination of bacterial specimens rather high powers of the microscope, and therefore also good illumination, are necessary. The latter is secured chiefly by condensing lenses placed between the mirror and the object. Immersion objectives have, over dry objectives, the double advantage of increasing illumination and diminishing the evils of refraction. Clearness and distinctness of the picture is as important as magnification. That microscope is of little value which shows "men as trees walking." Medium-power lenses may usually suffice for ordinary purposes, provided their definition be good. But for the highest class of work homogeneous immersion objectives, with strong and adjustable illuminating apparatus, are necessary.

Inoculation experiments upon animals serve several purposes. It is by this means that the truth of the germ theory of disease has been finally and fully proven. Inoculation experiments are the final steps in deciding for or against the specific causative agency of a particular germ. They afford, in otherwise doubtful or difficult cases, most valuable diagnostic in-

9

formation. They settle the questions of duration and
degree of virulence in germs of varying activity.
They are the crucial tests of specific preventive and
curative methods and agents, such as the antitoxin and
antitoxic treatment of diphtheria. Finally, they are
used to determine, with each infectious disease, the
various possible channels of infection.

Bacteria are inoculated on the skin, into and under
the skin, into the solid tissues and the body cavities.
They are introduced by feeding, by inhalation, and
even directly into the blood current. Thus, if the
supposed germs of erysipelas be under investigation,
they would be tested upon superficial wounds. Those
of cholera and typhoid fever would naturally be tried
by feeding; those of tuberculosis and suppuration by
all the methods. If we suspect that general miliary
tuberculosis is the result of an irruption of tubercular
material into a blood vessel, we may test the suspicion
by inoculations of tubercular cultures into the blood.
If we suspect the importance of a combination of non-
bacterial and bacterial factors in the production of a
disease, we may settle the question by experiments
with the former agents, then with the bacteria, and
then with both together. Such considerations reveal
the significance and value of inoculation experiments
in bacteriology, and their necessity in promoting its
beneficent work.

The history of bacteriology in its relation to practical medicine is similar to that of many other con-

tributions of science. Though its importance and value are now universally recognized, it is not many years since it was looked upon with some suspicion and even derision by many practitioners. Its place was thought to be in the experimental laboratory rather than in the consulting room. It was for the student of science, not for the student of disease. The same thing was said of the chemical and microscopic examination of the urine. A physician of this city has told the writer of hearing an eminent medical teacher of the last generation say that he could learn all that he wished to know about the urine by a study of the case and an appeal to his unaided senses. To-day the most unpretending doctor understands and constantly practices examinations for albumen, sugar, casts, and other abnormal urinary contents. There are many physicians still living and working who remember the advent of the clinical thermometer and the smile of incredulity with which it was generally received. The little instrument of thermometric accuracy was a pretty scientific toy, but of no practical value. Who could not detect the presence and judge sufficiently of the degree of fever by the sense of touch alone? To-day every physician carries the instrument in his pocket and uses it in almost every case. So it is proving of bacteriology. Those who, recognizing or being taught early its meaning, began to use it in everyday diagnosis, braving the harmless stigma of being theorists and unpractical, have now the pleasant satisfaction of recognition as pioneers not only of science, but of everyday practical medicine. That which often enables us to diagnose earlier, more accurately, and with more certainty than by any other means, such common diseases as tuberculosis, malaria and diphtheria, needs now no justification by him who applies it. He knows, and it is now gladly acknowledged, that he is exhibiting more than the interest and zeal of the scientist: he is applying the helpful art of the physician.

The number of diseases in which bacterial diagnosis is applicable in everyday work is not yet large, but fortunately it includes several of great practical importance. The details of procedure are now so fully set forth in the books on bacteriology, diagnosis and practice that an extensive discussion of them here would be out of place. A brief description of some of them may, however, be appropriate.

Acute specific urethritis usually declares itself so clearly in its symptoms and clinical history that bacterial diagnosis is seldom a necessity, though, being so simple and rapid, it may properly be applied in every suspected case. But in the presence of special circumstances or difficulties, clinical, medico-legal or social, it is of great value. The procedure is as follows: Having prepared the specimen upon the cover glass by the usual method of spreading, drying and heating, it is floated upon or covered with a cold watery solution of methyl blue. After one-half minute to two

minutes, according to the strength of the solution, it is
washed thoroughly in water, the clean side wiped dry,
and it is ready to examine. Under the microscope
the diplococci of gonorrhœa will be seen, in appearance much like two coffee beans, lying upon or in the
pus cells. They will be stained deep blue, while the
nuclei of the pus and epithelial cells are light blue.
The bacteria occur singly or in swarms, usually within
the cells, this being one of their striking characteristics. The protoplasm of the cells may be counter-
stained with an acid anilin dye, an alcoholic solution
of eosin, thus making the picture more striking and
the bacteria more conspicuous; but this is of no great
importance. As thus carried out, the procedure is
sufficient for all ordinary clinical purposes. But
since there are other bacteria, more or less closely resembling the gonococci, which may be found in the
same localities, examinations requiring medico-legal
accuracy must be carried further. The gonococci are
decolorized under the Gram method of staining.
They occur characteristically in groups within the
cells. They do not grow upon the ordinary culture
media, such as potato, beef gelatin, or beef-agar.
These tests having been applied the diagnosis becomes as nearly absolute as can be without culture
upon human blood serum and inoculations upon human beings.

The bacteriological diagnosis of diphtheria has a
special importance as a measure for the protection of

the public health and in view of the specific antitoxin
treatment. So true is this that in many cities, including our own, laboratories and trained examiners
are provided, at public expense, for doing this and
similar work. Many progressive practitioners also in
smaller communities are becoming skillful in thus
making the diagnosis. The microscope alone, while
often affording a high degree of probability to the ex-
pert diagnostician, is not thoroughly reliable, since
other bacilli, similar in appearance to those of diphtheria, may be found in the throat, or the specific microbes may be few and escape detection. Cultivations are therefore necessary, and, fortunately, are not
difficult.

The bacilli of diphtheria stain fairly well with simple watery solutions of the basic anilin dyes. They
are most perfectly colored with the Loeffler alcoholic
solution of methyl blue containing a very small per
cent. of potassium hydrate. As thus stained, they
appear as straight or slightly curved rods, the ends
usually more strongly colored than the center, and
often staining in segments somewhat resembling a
chain of micrococci. A striking feature of these bacilli is their variability of form, especially on different
culture media and in cultures or membranes of different ages.

Diphtheria bacilli grow most rapidly upon Loeffler's
culture medium, composed of three parts blood serum
and one part glucose-bouillon. In the incubator the

growth precedes that of other bacteria which may be present, often being recognizable in eight to twelve hours. A particle of this growth, removed from the tube and stained, reveals under the microscope the characteristic picture of the diphtheria bacilli. Scraping off with a sterilized wire or cotton swab a small amount of the membrane from the throat or other seat of disease, rubbing it onto the culture material, and placing the latter in the incubator, the diagnosis can usually be settled in twelve or at most twenty-four hours. Such cultures may also be made, though more slowly, by keeping the tubes in any warm place, as near a stove or furnace register, and upon any of the ordinary culture media. But for rapid diagnosis blood serum is necessary. Should questions arise as to the accuracy of such diagnosis or the virulence of the microbes, they may be settled by inoculations upon animals. The discovery of the specific diphtheria germ, and of methods of ready recognition, has resulted in establishing the fact that what has been called membranous croup is usually laryngeal diphtheria, and that there are many cases of exudative sore throat resembling diphtheria, some heretofore tentatively distinguished and some not, which are due to other causes. It therefore affords a welcome means of eliminating hitherto unavoidable uncertainty or error from reputable practice, and imposition from respectable charlatanism.

While the peculiar bodies found in the blood, and

commonly held to be the probable cause of malaria,
are not classified among the bacteria, yet their study is
so closely associated with bacteriology that reference
may properly be made to them here as in all recent
works on this subject. The malarial plasmodia are
protoplasmic bodies, varying in size and shape, often
pigmented, and to be found, most frequently during
or near the time of a paroxysm, in the blood of one
suffering from ague. They have not been successfully cultivated outside the body; final demonstration
of their character and specific causative agency is
therefore still lacking. Nevertheless they are so constantly associated with the disease, and in such a significant way, that their presence is now generally held
to afford ground for positive diagnosis, and therefore
for a clinical distinction between this and other diseases. Bedside experience is constantly confirming
this belief. In obscure cases the examination of the
blood has come to be relied upon by the highest clinical authorities. This examination, though at times
tedious, is not at all difficult. Puncture of the lobe
of the ear, or the finger, yields the droplet of blood,
which is transferred to the cover glass and immediately examined unstained. The blood specimen may
also be examined after staining with methyl blue, having first been simply mixed with the dye or dried and
heated by the ordinary method; or, much better, fixed
by prolonged heating or by immersion in equal parts
of alcohol and ether. Counter-staining may be done

with alcoholic eosin. Following the latter method, the blood cells are seen to be red, the bodies of the parasites blue, their nuclei colorless, and the nucleolus dark blue. Probably the most satisfactory plan is to examine the blood unstained.

Different varieties of plasmodia have been described as associated with the different types of malaria, but this question, as well as many others concerning the supposed malarial parasite, is still unsettled. Only the diagnostic value of the organism is generally agreed upon.

A number of diseases occurring only occasionally in man, the microbes of which are known, may be positively identified by bacteriological methods. Such are glanders, anthrax, and the ray-fungus disease, actinomycosis. In a larger number of disorders, of which pneumonia, cholera, erysipelas and tetanus are types, the identification of the bacteria is occasionally of diagnostic value, though usually such procedures are not called for. It is, however, possible, and with increasing frequency and value, where a well-equipped laboratory is available, to call bacteriology into service in the diagnosis of infectious or supposedly infectious diseases.

The character of several disorders, chiefly of the skin, caused by microscopic fungi belonging to the moulds or yeasts, may be established by the microscope or by artificial cultivation of the parasites. To this group belong ringworm, favus, and the brownish scaly skin disease, tinea versicolor.

The bacteria generally believed to be the cause of typhoid fever are so constantly associated in the excretions with others resembling them that they cannot be identified by microscopic examination nor by ordinary methods of cultivation. Bacteriology therefore does not, unfortunately, offer to the physician any direct means of diagnosis in this disease. But of late a procedure has come forward illustrating the indirect application of bacteriological diagnosis. It has been observed that if typhoid bacilli are brought into contact with the blood serum of one suffering from typhoid fever, they lose their motility and gather into swarms. This Widal test is applied as follows: A pure culture of typhoid bacilli being at hand, and having been examined to make certain that the bacilli show the normal motility, a particle of the culture is thoroughly mixed with distilled water, or, still better, a fresh culture is made in bouillon, and from this a few drops are taken. A drop of fresh blood or of dried blood moistened with distilled water is now added. From this mixture of typhoid bacilli and suspected blood a portion is transferred to a cover glass, the latter being immediately inverted over a concavity in a glass slide. The microscope now soon shows the bacilli gathering into swarms or clumps, and at the same time losing their motility. Should both of these phenomena occur, the reaction is said to be typical, and the inference is made that the blood came from one suffering from typhoid fever. The time re-

quired varies from a few minutes to half an hour or
more, the bacteria-containing fluid being meantime
protected against drying by vaselin or other adhesive
applied to the margin of the cover glass.

The specific character of this Widal reaction is still
under debate. Should it prove to be such, it will be
of great clinical value in this disease, and may open
the way to a similar diagnosis of other diseases whose
bacteria are known but are difficult of identification by
ordinary means.

A method of diagnosis closely associated with,
though neither originating from nor entirely depend-
ent upon bacteriology, is that by inoculation. Inoculation is frequently practiced as the final step in an
otherwise incomplete bacteriological demonstration,
but is sometimes sufficient of itself, and directly, to
establish a diagnosis. If in a suspicious case the discovery or identification of the bacteria be difficult or
impossible, inoculation of animals with material from
the suspected body may result in such an unmistakable attack of the disease as to remove all doubt. Or
such inoculation, with its resulting disease in the animal, may afford an easy opportunity for the discovery
and identification of the bacteria. Thus glanders,
rabies and tetanus in animals or human beings may
usually be certainly identified by inoculation of susceptible animals. By this method obscure cases of
tuberculosis, in which the bacilli are not easily found,
such as those involving the skin, glands, bones, joints,

intestinal canal and genito-urinary organs, may be
cleared up.

It is probably in tuberculosis that bacteriological
diagnosis has won its most striking and complete triumph. The frequency and seriousness of the disease,
and the importance of its early recognition, combine
to render this triumph the more noteworthy. It may
fairly be said that, by the skillful use of the means
now available, the diagnosis of tuberculosis, even in
its early and obscure forms, is almost completely com-
passed.

The microscopic identification of the tubercle bacillus is made possible by its almost peculiar staining
reaction. It stains only with difficulty, but, being
stained, resists decolorizing agents more than other
bacteria. To this rule there are but few exceptions,
and those, with care, readily recognized in ordinary
work. Many methods, differing in details, and all
based upon the rule just stated, have been devised for
staining the tubercle bacilli. But few of them are in
common use. In the original Koch-Ehrlich method
anilin oil was used as a mordant. Carbolic acid has
been found to answer a similar purpose. The staining solution now generally used is called Ziehl's carbol-fuchsin, being made as follows: To distilled water is added 5 per cent. of crystallized carbolic acid, 10
per cent. of alcohol, and 1 per cent. of dry fuchsin.
After complete solution of the solids, and filtration, it
is ready for use. Decolorization is accomplished by

20 to 30 per cent. solutions of nitric acid. As contrast color, methyl blue is used in watery solution. To hasten the process in everyday work the carbolfuchsin solution is applied hot, and to further save time the decolorizing and counter-staining are accomplished in one operation by combining the methyl blue and 25 per cent. sulphuric acid. In detail the process is as follows: Having spread the suspicious material upon cover glasses, dried and heated them, by the method already described, the dye is dropped upon the glass and the latter held by forceps over a clean flame until steam rises. If evaporation occur to dryness, more of the dye is added. A better method, though more wasteful of staining solution, is to heat the dye in a dish, floating the cover glasses upon the liquid. After two or three minutes' exposure to the dye, the glasses are rinsed in water, washed in the acid solution till the color fades out, then in alcohol for a few seconds to wash out the altered dye, and then thoroughly rinsed in water to remove the acid and alcohol. If examined at this stage the tubercle bacilli will be seen stained red, other bacteria being colorless. To counter-stain the specimen it is subjected for fifteen to thirty seconds to a watery solution of methyl blue, after which it is again rinsed in water. Inverted over a drop of distilled water and examined, the tubercle bacilli will be found still red, while other bacteria are blue. The whole process requires from three to five minutes. By this method

the bacilli are somewhat altered in shape, and perhaps do not resist strong decolorizing agents as well as those colored by a slower process. The best results are got by allowing the specimens to lie in the cold carbol-fuchsin for twelve hours or more. If the bacilli are few and therefore difficult to find, several methods are available for concentrating them. Pure liquid car-bolic acid added to sputum coagulates the parts most likely to contain the bacilli, thus rendering the selec-tion easier. If sputum be diluted with five or ten times its volume of water containing a small per cent. of potassium or sodium hydrate, and boiled, it be-comes liquefied and may be set aside for a day or two to settle in a conical glass. The sediment may now be examined with more certainty of finding the bacilli. Or the sputum, thus liquefied or simply shaken with water, may be rapidly precipitated with the centrifu-gal machine. The microscopic examination of the specimen thus prepared may at once reveal the tuber-cle bacilli, or may require great care and painstaking, involving considerable time and the study of a num-ber of specimens obtained at different times. Only positive results are of definite significance. The find-ing of tubercle bacilli stamps the case as tuberculosis. A negative result is only of relative significance, its value depending upon circumstances and upon the thoroughness and skill of the examination. It does not absolutely exclude tuberculosis, since the bacilli may not have been present in the material examined or may have been overlooked. Sections of tissue to be examined for tubercle bacilli are treated as follows: They are stained for about thirty minutes in carbol-fuchsin solution, washed for about one minute in 5 per cent. sulphuric acid, then for the same time in alcohol; they are then counter-stained for three or four minutes in weak methyl blue, again quickly washed in alcohol, immersed till clear in oil of cloves, and are ready to examine in Canada balsam.

It is to be remembered that the successful identification of the tubercle bacilli requires that the material shall come from the seat of disease, shall contain the bacteria, and that the examination shall have been properly made. Failure of any of these requirements will necessarily yield but negative results. Fortunately, there remain two other available tests, the one the inoculation of susceptible animals, already referred to, the other the diagnostic injection of tuberculin.

The tuberculin injection is, like the Widal test for typhoid fever and the Mallein injection for the detection of glanders, an illustration of indirect bacteriological diagnosis. In 1890 Koch announced the discovery, in the culture-products of tubercle bacilli, of a substance which, being injected into animals or men suffering from tuberculosis, would produce certain local and constitutional reactions and, as he then thought, curative effects. Hopes thus raised in the latter direction have not been fulfilled, for reasons

which Koch himself has recently admitted and explained. But the diagnostic significance of the tuberculin injection remains. Until recently this
method has, except in the hands of a few experimenters, been restricted to the diagnosis of the disease in
animals. Here its value and reliability are now generally recognized by veterinarians. It is hardly too
much to say that to-day the efforts for the eradication
of tuberculosis among cattle and for the protection of
the public against tuberculous meat and milk center
about the tuberculin diagnosis. Of late the profession has been recovering from the fear of harm by this
procedure, and on good grounds. The dangers have
certainly been much exaggerated. The hypodermic
injection of from one-half to three milligrams of tuberculin will usually produce, in a person having any
form of tuberculosis, a recognizable reaction sufficient
to establish the diagnosis. The pulse quickens, the
temperature rises, and there is more or less accompanying local and general disturbance, all of which
subside within a few hours or days. In order that
the results may be correctly interpreted and possible
dangers avoided, certain precautions and preparations
are necessary. The tuberculin must be genuine and
not too old. It must have been proven free from contamination, and should, if possible, have been previously tested upon a known case of tuberculosis.
The patient's pulse and temperature should have been
recorded at regular intervals for several days, and a

careful physical examination should have been made. Evidence of cerebral or renal tuberculosis should exclude this method of diagnosis, and in all cases violent reactions are unnecessary and should be avoided. With these precautions the tuberculin injection promises to become a valuable aid in the definite recognition of the disease in those early or obscure cases in which the other means of diagnosis are not available. The immediate future will doubtless bring the solution of some questions as yet unsettled concerning this method. If it shall be settled that the tuberculin reaction, properly induced, is a specific one, and limited to tuberculosis, and that the supposed dangers may, by its skillful use, be practically eliminated, we shall indeed be in a position to reaffirm the statement heretofore ventured: that the diagnostic problem of tuberculosis has been solved, and another contribution made by bacteriology to practical medicine.

XI.

NON-BACTERIAL FACTORS IN INFECTIOUS DISEASES.

THE writer has for some years past had much to say upon the subject of bacteriology and the germ theory of disease. He has also, largely by reason of circumstances, often been called upon to act as its special sponsor and defender. In so doing he has always recognized, and as opportunity offered has emphasized, the danger of a one-sided view which would overlook the other factors in the causation of the infectious diseases.

This danger, however, does not chiefly threaten those whose interest in bacteriology and opportunities for its study have led to a somewhat thorough knowledge, but rather the contrary. It might, I think, fairly be said that those whose interest in and study of bacteriology have led to something of a reputation as bacteriologists, are, for example, not as much troubled over the influence of a debauch in causing the drunkard's pneumonia as are many others over the question of the role of bacteria in this disease.

The writer has, therefore, for some time had in mind to prepare a paper upon the subject announced,

whose purpose should be, standing upon the double
ground of bacteriologist and clinician, to consider
some of the non-bacterial factors in diseases caused by
bacteria. Such a paper may serve, and is intended to
serve, in some sense as a culmination of the series prepared for the State Medical Society. By such a paper, too, he hopes to aid in reconciling bacteriology
and clinical medicine by showing that a beautiful harmony exists between them.

There are two classes of physicians to whom an address of this nature might be directed as a special plea:

First, there are some, a diminishing company, who,
by reason of grossly defective knowledge and equally
gross misunderstanding of bacteriologists, have con-
ceived a pronounced and outspoken antagonism, even
amounting to scoffing, against the germ explanation
of disease. They love to hurl such epithets as bacteria-maniac, but they never dare to allow themselves
to be inoculated with cultures of anthrax or tubercle
bacilli. From such men emanate the furious anti-
microbic articles which occasionally appear in medical
publications, the best answer to which is the fact that
no well-informed man answers them at all.

Second, there are those who, being intelligent and
competent physicians, are yet perplexed with many
doubts in regard to the germ theory of disease because
they cannot reconcile it with the facts of clinical medicine. They recognize the meaning of the general
acceptance of the theory, and feel the force of its sin-

ple logic. They fall in with the advancing current of opinion and conviction, and conscientiously obey its impulses. But they cannot just tell why they are where they are, or whither they and we are drifting. Possibly some of us who have had much to say to them about bacteriology have so frightened and confused them that they are unable to see that, though sometimes in the midst of foaming billows, they are nevertheless floating on a clear and beautiful stream of truth, and therefore need have no fear of their destiny. They will in time see that ancient landmarks are only for the time being somewhat obscured, somewhat changed, by the new view. To such I hope to say a helpful word, by showing the fact and method of a harmony between bacteriology and clinical medicine.

And first a few words toward a mutual understanding:

I am to deal with the non-bacterial factors in the infectious diseases; yet I shall have something to say about such things as numbers and virulence of bacteria as influencing infection. By the words "non-bacterial factors" is therefore meant agencies other than the mere presence of bacteria which influence the development of the infectious diseases.

As to the degree to which such factors influence particular infections, and the degree of importance to be attached to them in clinical medicine, I have not now much to say. The subject is of the greatest moment, but is out of place here, since this is a study of pathology, not of practice.

I shall assume two propositions to be true. First, that the infectious diseases, have, as their prime and essential cause, living poisons, commonly called germs, bacteria, microbes, and that without them these diseases do not exist. Second, that many agencies other than the mere presence and growth of bacteria influence the development of the infectious diseases, even to the extent of assuming the role at times of controlling factors. Can these two propositions be harmonized? It is the chief purpose of this address to show that they can, by showing that the non-bacterial factors influence the development of the infectious diseases because they influence the growth of bacteria in the body. And so the whole matter comes down to a proposition which may be expressed in the simple analogy from agriculture, thus: Crops of grain are the products primarily and essentially of certain seeds; all other factors influence the production of grain crops by contribution to the growth of those seeds. So infectious diseases are primarily and essentially the products of the growth of disease seeds or germs; all other factors influence their development by contribution to the growth of those germs in the body. But, let me repeat, and be it remembered, this is the statement for pathological, not necessarily for clinical guidance. The agriculturist would not misinterpret his part of the analogy; neither need the physician misinterpret his.

We all recognize that there have been many fanciful explanations of the infectious diseases, many things fancifully invoked as factors in their causation. But we all also recognize that even long before the identification of disease germs various agencies, non-bacterial in character, were shown to be closely associated with and even to play a part in the production of these maladies. The importance of these agencies has been seen to vary in different diseases and under differing conditions, being sometimes but slight, sometimes seeming to stand in the foreground as exciting or predisposing causes. But the fact of their importance and influence has been and is unquestioned and unquestionable.

For example, no one asserts or believes that other factors than the peculiar poison, except possibly age, play an important role either as exciting or predisposing causes of measles. But it is commonly and strongly believed that the tubercle bacilli by no means stand alone in the development of tuberculosis. Every one recognizes, after the experience of recent years, that the disease called la grippe, in its epidemic form, attacks many without the aid of recognizable predisposing causes. But every one also knows that acute pneumonia seldom comes by infection alone.

Granting that the infectious diseases are, in the last

analysis, due to the growth of bacteria in the body, the questions arise: What other agencies enter into their production, and what role do such other factors play? Can the facts of clinical experience and the facts of laboratory work be harmonized?

I believe that in large measure they may. And, further, if one will but observe closely, it will be found that laboratory experiment in this direction has confirmed many of the facts of clinical experience, has furnished a more correct interpretation of others, and has thrown light upon almost all. When we come to study the factors other than the mere presence of bacteria which enter into infection, we find that they fall into two groups, one relating to the persons infected, the other to the bacteria. What now are some of these factors, and to what extent has bacteriology increased our knowledge of their importance and meaning?

First, race. It has long been observed that certain races of men seem less susceptible to certain infections than others. For instance, the negro is believed to be less susceptible to yellow fever than the white. Can we find confirmation of such a principle in the bacteriological laboratory? We do find many. Thus the rat is comparatively unsusceptible to anthrax, while the guinea pig readily succumbs to small dosage. Algerian sheep resist anthrax strongly, while ordinary sheep easily fall a prey to this serious disease. Hens and frogs have a natural immunity against anthrax, and white mice against glanders. Dosage and other conditions being the same, white rats yield to infection with anthrax most readily, gray rats next, and black rats least. Many more examples might be given illustrating the principle that the growth of disease germs may be more or less influenced by the race or species of animal infected.

Second, just as race seems to play a part in the infectious diseases, so does age. For instance, very young infants seem to possess a relative insusceptibility to measles and scarlatina; later their vulnerability increases, and again seems to decline with advancing years.

The same thing may be demonstrated in the laboratory. It is a general rule, well known to bacteriological experimenters, that young animals are more readily infected with cultures of bacteria than are the old. Certain animals, which at a mature age show a strong degree of immunity against a disease, may be comparatively easily inoculated in early life. In this respect also, therefore, experiments with bacteria confirm the observations at the bedside.

Third. Into the production of individual susceptibility many and various factors enter, some of which we understand, while others are still mysteries. Some are general, others local in action. Thus it has long been observed that persons suffering from diabetes mellitus are specially prone to the development of suppuration and tuberculosis; that erysipelas commonly follows a wound, and that distinct traumatism is almost invariably the antecedent of non-tubercular subcutaneous abscess.

Many experiments, some of them of a most ingenious character, have been made to solve the problems of individual susceptibility, general and local. A few of these may be cited:

The facts quoted in regard to diabetes being so conspicuous, suggested lines of experiment which have proven most interesting and significant. Thus if white mice are rendered artificially diabetic by feeding with phloridzine, they at once become susceptible to glanders bacilli, which, naturally, they strongly resist. The ordinary pus microbes are, in small quantities, ordinarily without much effect when introduced under the skin of rats; but if associated with a solution of sugar, suppuration is much more likely to occur. Animals not susceptible to the disease called symptomatic anthrax (black leg) may be successfully inoculated with these bacilli provided the animals are at the same time injected with lactic acid.

Clinical experience indicates that many agencies having a more or less general effect upon the body predispose to infection, and there are definite bacteriological experiments confirming the belief. Certain animals fed on certain kinds of food are more susceptible to anthrax than when otherwise nourished. Starvation renders pigeons much more easily infected with the same bacilli. Anthrax and some other bac-

teria have been shown to develop more certainly in
animals after great fatigue. Pus microbes, anthrax
bacilli, and other microbes, have been found to infect
with more certainty and violence certain animals in
which an artificial anemia has been produced by
bleeding. One of Pasteur's classical experiments con-
sisted in rendering hens, ordinarily unsusceptible, susceptible to anthrax by artificial cooling of their
bodies; and conversely, artificial elevation of the temperature of frogs has changed their natural immunity
into susceptibility to anthrax. A similar result has
been shown to follow in animals deprived of water.
Thus many of the things included under the general
term bad hygiene have been definitely shown to render animals more susceptible to the growth of bacteria.

Previous disease, as shown by clinical experience
and by definite bacteriological experiment, may predispose to subsequent infection, though this agency is
most often seen to act as a local rather than a general
predisposing factor.

Local, like general predisposition, may be brought
about by an indefinite number and variety of things
which temporarily or permanently injure the tissues.
Here belong traumatisms, local inflammations, antecedent local or general diseases which produce distinct
local injury, and serious alterations in the local circulation of the blood.

The result of all such agencies is a locus minoris
resistentiæ, a point of lessened resistance to the en-

trance and growth of bacteria. The broken skin not only more readily admits bacteria, but the injured tissue less easily resists their growth.

The poison of measles does not produce either whooping cough or tuberculosis, but the respiratory mucous membranes, altered and damaged by measles, fall a more ready prey to the next invaders.

The inhalation of metallic or other dust cannot of itself produce more than a simple inflammation with resulting fibrosis. But it may open the way for the entrance and growth of tubercle bacilli.

Some of the most beautiful of bacteriological experiments have been made to test this matter of local lessened resistance. It may be interesting to quote a few of these experiments.

Bacteria injected into the circulation do not often attach themselves to the heart valves, neither does a direct aseptic injury of the valves, as by a clean needle, produce ulcerative endocarditis. In other words, simple injury, or the mere presence of bacteria, do not necessarily result in ulcerative endocarditis. But let the valves be deliberately injured, and about the same time let suppurative bacteria be introduced into the blood current, and these bacteria will be found lodged and growing at the point of lessened resistance. A blow over the tibia without break of the skin does not result in subcutaneous or subperiosteal abscess. But experiment has repeatedly shown that such simple injuries, which, if not infected, remain non-suppurative, are very likely to suppurate or show other infection if the simultaneous presence of bacteria be assured. Wandering bacteria are likely to lodge at such a spot, just as vultures are to alight upon carrion.

Other interesting experiments have been made showing that the introduction of aseptic irritants together with bacteria into the tissues or directly into the circulation is much more likely to be followed by the lodgment and growth of the bacteria than when the latter are introduced alone. And thus in all directions the old doctrine of local and general susceptibility to infection is confirmed and illuminated, while at the same time the specific causative agency of the bacteria remains unquestioned.

But not only do agencies affecting the body influence infection. Certain considerations concerning the bacteria themselves are of great importance. Here, too, clinical experience and laboratory experiment agree.

Two children being exposed to apparently the same degree to measles, one takes the disease while the other does not. One child has virulent scarlatina or diphtheria, while others in the same community have but mild attacks. At one time a mild type of scarlatina prevails, as in this community during recent years; at another we have to confront what a venerable practitioner among us has described as the dying kind.

Let us see, now, leaving out of consideration questions of susceptibility affecting the body, how far bacteriology has thrown light upon these problems.

We expose, in an ordinary room, a series of culture plates; after a time they are placed in an incubator, and some are found to be infected with the microbes of erysipelas, suppuration, tuberculosis, or diphtheria, while others remain sterile or show only ordinary non-pathogenic bacteria. The microbes have, in the terse phrase of Welch, hit some and missed others. Imagine now these plates to be living persons, and we at once see one reason why, among a number seemingly similarly exposed, some are attacked while others escape.

Again examining our plates, we shall see another significant fact: Some have developed but few colonies, while others show many. In a word, some have been hit by many microbes, others by but few; hence upon some a more pronounced growth than others. Here, too, therefore, we see, in the number of bacteria which fall upon the soil, a second possible explanation of our problems. More direct experiment has abundantly shown that the inference just suggested is correct. Let a series of similar lesions be infected with bacteria taken from the same culture, but in varying numbers, and, other things being equal, it will be found that those lesions entertaining the larger number of microbes are more likely to be successfully infected, and in a ratio of probability increasing with

the number of bacteria. This is more readily clinically recognized with those diseases, and experiment-
ally with those bacteria, susceptibility to which in the
animals experimented with is not great.

And thus we have established the bacteriological
doctrine that the number of bacteria in an important
way influences infection, confirming the clinical doctrine that quantity of poison and great exposure have
much to do in determining the development of an infectious disease.

Examining our culture plates again, we may discover a third phenomenon: Upon some of these
plates the germs of diphtheria have fallen. We make
inoculation experiments and find that some of these
diphtheria bacilli are of great virulence, others produce but mild results, while others cannot be made to
produce either typical lesions or general symptoms of
diphtheria. Inoculating animals with these various
types of diphtheria bacilli, we find that some produce
pronounced local lesions with equally pronounced
constitutional symptoms. Evidently these germs possess their full biological characteristics. Others produce fairly typical local lesions, but little or no constitutional disturbance, while others cause but slight
local disturbance. Yet these are all genuine diphtheria bacilli. Evidently they differ biologically in
this, that some are possessed of their full powers, others are weakened, while some have lost all or almost
all pathogenic property. And this is the reason for
the different effects upon the inoculated animals.

And thus we become impressed with a third truth: that the virulence of the microbes plays an important role, not only in the typical development of an infectious disease, but in the violence of the local and general disturbance.

That personal immunity or susceptibility and variations in number and virulence of bacteria are often, indeed usually, intricately combined is evident. So true is this that the clinical evidence of the non-bacterial factors in infectious diseases is often difficult to sift. We must turn to experiment upon animals for a solution of many of the problems. The answer which bacteriology has to give has, it is hoped, been partly set forth. More might be said, but surely enough has been brought out to show that clinical medicine and modern bacteriology are not and need not be out of harmony. And he who has a clear view of both will be in no danger of being either a bacteria-maniac or a bacteria-phobic.

A word in conclusion, and a simple illustration and analogy. The more closely these things are studied the more clear does it become that we have in bacteriology but another example of some very old truths.

There is an ancient parable which tells us that a sower went forth to sow, and as he sowed some seed fell by the wayside, some upon stony ground, and some upon good soil, with the result that some failed entirely, some grew but faintly, while some flourished. In the simple and stately scriptural phrase is set forth the universally recognized truth of agriculture, that other factors than the seeds have to do with the gathering of a harvest. The sun must shine, the rain must fall, and the soil must be suitable, or the harvest will not come. Yet what agriculturist so simple-minded as not to know that for a harvest of corn or wheat he must plant the seeds of corn or wheat?

Does one imagine that catching cold causes pneumonia? Then let him also assert that sunshine produces wheat. Does he assert that bad water causes typhoid fever? Then let him also assert that rain causes oats. Does he believe that weak lungs degenerate and develop tuberculosis? Then let him also assert that the soil of the earth produces corn.

Is anyone perplexed when told that the germs of diphtheria and pneumonia may sometimes be found in the throats of healthy persons, and in the absence of active disease? And does he therefore doubt the specific causative agency of these bacteria or of all bacteria? Let him, in the words of the poet, go out to commune with nature. She will indeed speak to him a varied language. Let him study the ground in the winter, observing the various seeds scattered in and upon the soil, yet producing no plants. Then let him watch and see what occurs with the advent of spring, with its sunshine and warmth. The seeds sprout and grow, and the plant springs up; not because of the moisture and heat, but because these prepared the way for the one thing essential, the seed.

Without the proper seed, the most fertile soil under the most favorable conditions produces no corn, no wheat. Without the specific germs the body suffers from no typhoid, no diphtheria, no tuberculosis.

This simple, illuminating analogy between agriculture and bacteriology I would leave as the last thought with him who reads these pages. If he will bear it in mind, he will seldom be at loss to understand the germ theory of disease and many of the problems arising out of it. It will make him a better and a clearer thinker about disease. And, being a clearer thinker, he will be a more efficient actor as a physician.

When once he has seen, what every agriculturist sees, that sunshine and rain and soil and seed must work together to produce the harvest, then he will see how germs may be the direct exciting cause of the infectious diseases, into whose production, however, many other factors enter, and often play an important part. And then he will see the beautiful harmony between clinical medicine and bacteriology, one truth only aiding another.

www.ingramcontent.com/pod-product-compliance
Lightning Source LLC
Chambersburg PA
CBHW021810190326
41518CB00007B/536